BSAVA Pocketbook for Veterinary Nurses

second edition

Editor:
Emma Gerrard

**DipHE(CVN) DipAVN(Small Animal)
BSc(Hons)CVN RVN**

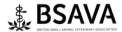

BSAVA
BRITISH SMALL ANIMAL VETERINARY ASSOCIATION

Published by:

British Small Animal Veterinary Association
Woodrow House, 1 Telford Way, Waterwells Business Park, Quedgeley,
Gloucester GL2 2AB

A Company Limited by Guarantee in England
Registered Company No. 2837793
Registered as a Charity

ISBN 978-1-910443-88-0

The publishers, editors and contributors cannot take responsibility for
information provided on dosages and methods of application of drugs
mentioned or referred to in this publication. Details of this kind must
be verified in each case by individual users from up to date literature
published by the manufacturers or suppliers of those drugs. Veterinary
surgeons are reminded that in each case they must follow all
appropriate national legislation and regulations (for example, in the
United Kingdom, the prescribing cascade) from time to time in force.

Printed by Zenith Media, Pontypool NP4 0DQ
Printed on ECF paper made from sustainable forests.

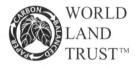

WORLD
LAND
TRUST™

www.carbonbalancedpaper.com
CBP021925

Carbon Balancing is delivered by World Land Trust, an international
conservation charity, who protects the world's most biologically
important and threatened habitats acre by acre. Their Carbon
Balanced Programme offsets emissions through the purchase and
preservation of high conservation value forests.

19135PUBS23

Contents

- **Foreword** v
- **Preface** vi
- **A few notes on using this book** vii

A
- Anaesthetic agents 1
- Anaesthetic checklists 7
- Anaesthetic emergencies 10
- Anaesthetic equipment 16
- ASA physical status and classifications scale 31

B
- Bandaging 32
- Biochemistry reference ranges 41
- Blood cell types 42
- Blood collection tubes 44
- Blood pressure measurement 46
- Blood pressure values for dogs and cats 54
- Blood sampling 55
- Blood smear preparation 63
- Blood staining procedures 66
- Blood transfusion 67
- Body condition scoring scheme – cats 86
- Body condition scoring scheme – dogs 88
- Body condition scoring scheme – rabbits 90

C
- Calculating blood loss 92
- Cleaning the operating theatre 95
- Clinical audits 97

D
- Dental recording chart – cat 98
- Dental recording chart – dog 99

E
- Ear cytology 101
- Electrocardiography 104

F
- Faecal examination 107
- Feeding tube selection 108
- Feeding tubes – nursing considerations 112
- Fine needle aspiration of a mass 114
- Fluid therapy 116
- Folding gowns and drapes 120

G
- Gowning and gloving 122

H
- Haematology reference ranges 127
- Hair and skin sampling procedures 128
- Hand hygiene 135

I
- Infection control 137
- Intravenous catheter management 139

L
- Laboratory samples – packaging for external analysis 143

■ **M**
- Mucous membrane colour — 147
- Muscle condition scoring scheme – cats — 148
- Muscle condition scoring scheme – dogs — 150

■ **O**
- Opioids — 153

■ **P**
- Packed cell volume – how to perform a PCV — 155
- Pain assessment — 158
- Pain scoring – cat — 162
- Pain scoring – dog — 164
- Pain scoring – rabbit — 166
- Patient assessment – daily tasks — 168
- Patient assessment – routine parameters — 169
- Physiotherapy — 170
- PROTECT ME — 172

■ **R**
- Radiographic film faults — 175
- Radiographic positioning — 177
- Radiographic positioning – advanced — 204
- Recumbent patient care — 211
- Resting energy requirement (RER) calculation — 213

■ **S**
- Scrubbing — 215
- Sterilization – packing instruments — 219
- Sterilization indicators — 221
- Surgical checklist — 222
- Sutures — 224

■ **T**
- Temperature conversion — 231
- Theatre – maintenance of asepsis — 232
- Total solids – using a refractometer — 234

■ **U**
- Urinalysis — 236
- Urinary catheters – cats — 238
- Urinary catheters – dogs — 240
- Urine specific gravity (USG) normal values — 248

■ **V**
- Vernier scale — 249
- Vital signs – normal ranges in common species — 250

■ **W**
- Wound drain management — 251
- Wound dressings — 252
- Wound recognition and treatment — 258

■ **References** — 263
■ **Emergency doses** — 264

Foreword

I feel very honoured to write the foreword for the second edition of the *BSAVA Pocketbook for Veterinary Nurses*. Veterinary nurses are an integral part of the veterinary team. Nurses, with their specific skills, knowledge and empathy, are vital to the patients' welfare whilst under veterinary care. Animals are more likely to get better, and get better faster, if they have good nursing care. This book is packed with the sort of information that allows nurses to deliver that care. It is presented in a format that makes it easy to carry around, but it will find its home at the heart of the clinic.

The editor and production team behind this publication have worked hard to make it as relevant and practical as possible. BSAVA and its increasing nurse membership owe them a debt of gratitude and I would like to thank them all for their efforts.

Ian Ramsey

BVSc PhD DSAM DipECVIM-CA FHEA FRCVS
BSAVA President (2020–2021)

Preface

It is my honour to introduce the second edition of the *BSAVA Pocketbook for Veterinary Nurses*. This edition aims to build on the legacy that Louise O'Dwyer began in 2012. It includes extracts from the first edition and some additional material in a new full colour and alphabetical format. The pocketbook is designed as a 'quick reference' guide to offer essential, practical and easily accessible information in a concise design.

I would like to thank the BSAVA for their continued support, and in particular the Publications team for their help and guidance when preparing this pocketbook. I would also like to acknowledge the BSAVA authors and editors whose work has been gathered for inclusion in this pocketbook.

All feedback is welcome at **publications@bsava.com**.

In memory of Louise O'Dwyer.

Emma Gerrard
DipHE(CVN) DipAVN(Small Animal) BSc(Hons)CVN RVN

October 2020

Emma qualified as a Veterinary Nurse in 2005 from Myerscough College, Preston. She gained the Diploma of Higher Education Clinical Veterinary Nursing in June 2009, followed by the RCVS Diploma in Advanced Veterinary Nursing in January 2010. In 2011, she graduated from the BSc (Hons) Clinical Veterinary Nursing top-up degree. Emma works at an independent general mixed practice in Powys and locums for Vets Now. Her interests are very varied and include infection control and surgical nursing. Emma began volunteering in 2013 for the BVNA as Regional Representative and for the BSAVA Cymru/Wales Region. She has been a member of the Membership Development Committee, and a member and Treasurer of the Cymru/Wales Committee. Emma is a companion and farm animal RAMA, a clinical coach, article writer for several veterinary nursing publications, and a tutor for ONCORE ePD.

A few notes on using this book

- This book is designed to condense the common nursing procedures into one pocket-sized book that can be carried around easily in a tunic or scrub top pocket.
- It contains much of the basic information on certain procedures; for more detailed information a more in-depth text should be consulted.
- All procedures should be carried out under the direction of a veterinary surgeon; veterinary nurses should ensure they carry out these procedures under the remit of Schedule 3 of the Veterinary Surgeons Act 1966 (Part 1, paragraphs 6 and 7).
- Selected drugs are listed by generic name.
- All medications should be administered under the direction of a veterinary surgeon.
- A veterinary nurse should always refer to other source material if they are not familiar with the procedures mentioned in this guide.
- All sources used in this guide are referenced by a superscript number which refers to a bibliography at the back of the book.

NOTES

Anaesthetic agents [1, 5, 13]

Anaesthetic agents — intravenous

Steroids

- Alfaxalone

  Usage and effects
  - Alfaxan contains 10 mg/ml of alfaxalone. It is available in Australia, New Zealand and the UK. Because it does not contain Cremophor EL it can be used in dogs as well as cats for the induction and maintenance of anaesthesia.

  Contraindications and warnings
  - It must be injected slowly to avoid respiratory depression and resultant apnoea.

Dissociative anaesthetic agents

Produce a light plane of anaesthesia along with profound analgesia. The animal appears dissociated from its surroundings and procedures being carried out.

- Ketamine

  Usage and effects
  - Used on its own and in various combinations with alpha-2 agonists, opiate analgesics and benzodiazepines to produce anaesthesia in dogs, cats, rabbits and other exotics.

  Contraindications and warnings
  - Not suitable for use in animals with impaired renal function or hepatic function.

- Tiletamine

  Usage and effects
  - Similar to ketamine.
  - Available premixed with zolazepam (a benzo-diazepine) in USA and Australia.

Substituted phenols

- Propofol

  Usage and effects
  - Marketed as a milky white emulsion in soya bean oil, egg phosphatide and glycerol.

- Intravenous injection results in a rapid induction of anaesthesia which, if not maintained with an inhalation agent or further boluses of propofol, lasts about 15–20 minutes.
- Rapidly metabolized in the liver and elsewhere in the body. Animals with impaired liver function are less likely to experience prolonged recoveries when given propofol.
- Because of its rapid metabolism, it is non-cumulative and can be used as a maintenance anaesthetic agent. When used for this purpose, it is often delivered as a constant-rate infusion using a syringe driver.
- Does not produce prolonged anaesthesia in Greyhounds and other sighthounds.

Contraindications and warnings

- Some individuals develop severe muscle twitches after prolonged use.
- Following intravenous injection, a transient fall in blood pressure and cardiac output is seen along with a brief period of apnoea.
- The cardiovascular effects of propofol are at least as profound as those seen with thiopental.
- Propofol's main advantage over thiopental is its short duration of action and extra-hepatic metabolism. It is not a 'safer' anaesthetic even though it is often sold to owners as such.
- Most solutions do not contain preservatives but there are some available that do; thus care must be taken to adhere to disposal advice for individual products.

NOTES

Pharmacology of injectable agents

Drug	Routes of administration	Cardiovascular system effects	Respiratory system effects	Formulation and preparation
Alfaxalone	i.v. i.m. (unlicensed)	Myocardial depression associated with a compensatory increase in heart rate	Respiratory depression, may cause apnoea after injection	Alfaxalone is solubilized in a cyclodextrin that does not cause histamine release; can be used in cats and dogs
Ketamine	i.v. i.m.	Stimulates the sympathetic nervous system, increases heart rate, minimal effects on cardiac output	Minimal effects on the respiratory system, may cause an apneustic breathing pattern	Preparation contains a preservative
Propofol	i.v.: does not cause thrombophlebitis if injected outside the vein	Myocardial depression, vasodilation and bradycardia	Respiratory depression, may cause apnoea after injection	Propofol solubilized in egg phosphatide and soya bean oil, with or without benzyl alcohol as a preservative

Anaesthetic agents — volatile

Drug	Minimum alveolar concentration (%)	Solubility coefficient (blood/gas)	Maximum legal occupational exposure limits (ppm)
Isoflurane	Dog 1.28 Cat 1.63 Rabbit 2.05	1.5	50
Sevoflurane	Dog 2.1–2.36 Cat 2.58 Rabbit 3.7	0.68	60
Desflurane	Dog 7.2 Cat 9.8 Rabbit 5.7–7.1	0.42	–

Isoflurane
Usage and effects
- Less soluble than halothane and therefore produces even more rapid induction of and recovery from anaesthesia.
- Can be used as both induction and maintenance agent.
- Very useful for induction of anaesthesia in small mammals.
- Does not sensitize heart to adrenaline as much as halothane and so causes fewer cardiac arrhythmias.
- More potent respiratory depressant than halothane.

Contraindications and warnings
- Produces less severe myocardial depression than halothane (but overall fall in blood pressure is similar, due to more profound peripheral vasodilation).

Pharmacological characteristics
- Pungent smell and irritant to airways: animals may resent induction.
- Dose-dependent respiratory and cardiovascular system depression.

- Reduces systemic vascular resistance, leading to vasodilation and compensatory increase in heart rate.
- Little liver metabolism; most excreted via respiratory system at end of anaesthesia.
- Minimal effect on liver blood flow.

Sevoflurane
Usage and effects
- Less soluble still than isoflurane so rapid induction of and recovery from anaesthesia as well as rapid changes in anaesthetic depth.
- Depresses myocardial contractility (strength of heart's contractions) – similar to isoflurane, as is degree of peripheral vasodilation produced.
- Does not sensitize heart to adrenaline to the extent that halothane does so causes fewer arrhythmias.

Contraindications and warnings
- Rapid recoveries from anaesthesia can expose poor analgesic techniques – animals can wake up quickly and vocalize in pain. This must not be dismissed as dysphoria or 'a reaction to the anaesthetic'.
- Reacts with dry soda lime to produce 'Compound A' – a chemical known to be toxic to rats. It is not toxic to dogs in concentrations found during clinical use and sevoflurane can be used with circuits containing soda lime in dogs.

Pharmacological characteristics
- Odourless, non-irritant.
- Agent of choice for induction.
- Dose-dependent reduction in myocardial contractility and mean arterial blood pressure.
- Very little liver metabolism; rapidly excreted via lungs.

Desflurane
Usage and effects
- Very volatile (is nearly boiling at room temperature) and must be delivered using special electronically controlled vaporizer/blender.

IIII▶

- The least soluble of all the volatile agents and so produces the most rapid induction and recovery.

Contraindications and warnings
- Not yet in common use in veterinary practice.

Pharmacological characteristics
- Pungent smell; despite low blood solubility, rarely used for induction.
- Dose-dependent myocardial and respiratory system depression.
- Heart rate may increase due to stimulation of sympathetic nervous system.
- Very little liver metabolism; rapidly excreted via lungs.

NOTES

Anaesthetic checklists[16]

The use of safety checklists has become increasingly popular over recent years. The aim of these checklists is not only to prompt everyone involved in the process of anaesthetizing a patient to check that all equipment is present and correct, but also to improve dialogue amongst the whole team. This was highlighted by the World Health Organization's Safe Surgery Saves Lives initiative, in its attempt to reduce the number of surgical deaths worldwide. This initiative was first published in 2008 and has now been widely adopted.

The Association of Veterinary Anaesthetists (AVA) has produced a checklist and an implementation manual (ava.eu.com/resources/checklists). Each of the steps involved in the checklist has been included to reduce the risk of significant harm to the patient; it is not designed to be a comprehensive list of actions involved with anaesthetizing a patient. The idea is that it is not just a box ticking exercise; rather, it is the performance of the associated actions and the communication and information sharing that it promotes which is important.

Safety checklists should form part of the wider anaesthetic record for the patient and be saved in paper form or scanned electronically on to the patient's records.

A checklist is completed for every procedure at three specific time points:

- Pre-induction
- Pre-procedure
- Recovery.

Pre-induction checklist

The pre-induction checklist includes confirmation of:

- Patient name, owner consent and procedure
- Intravenous cannula in place and patent
- Airway equipment available and checked to be

functioning (including additional equipment, i.e. dog urinary catheter, if difficult airway suspected)
- Endotracheal tube cuffs checked
- Anaesthetic machine checked
- Adequate oxygen supply for the procedure
- Breathing system connected, checked and the adjustable pressure-limiting (APL) valve open
- Dedicated person assigned to monitor the patient
- Risks identified and communicated to all members of the team
- Emergency interventions available.

Pre-procedure checklist

The pre-procedure checklist includes confirmation of:

- Patient name and procedure
- Appropriate depth of anaesthesia
- Safety concerns communicated – this is another point at which any concerns regarding the patient should be aired to the whole team; an intervention plan should be made, if necessary, at this point.

Recovery checklist

The recovery checklist includes confirmation of:

- Safety concerns:
  - Airway
  - Breathing
  - Fluid balance
  - Body temperature
  - Pain
- Assessment and intervention plan
- Analgesia plan
- Person assigned to monitor patient.

Anaesthetic Safety Checklist

ASSOCIATION OF VETERINARY ANAESTHETISTS

Pre-Induction

- ☐ Patient NAME, owner CONSENT & PROCEDURE confirmed
- ☐ IV CANNULA placed & patent
- ☐ AIRWAY EQUIPMENT available & functioning
- ☐ Endotracheal tube CUFFS checked
- ☐ ANAESTHETIC MACHINE checked today
- ☐ Adequate OXYGEN for proposed procedure
- ☐ BREATHING SYSTEM connected, leak free & APL VALVE OPEN
- ☐ Person assigned to MONITOR patient
- ☐ RISKS identified & COMMUNICATED
- ☐ EMERGENCY INTERVENTIONS available

Pre-Procedure — Time Out

- ☐ Patient NAME & PROCEDURE confirmed
- ☐ DEPTH of anaesthesia appropriate
- ☐ SAFETY CONCERNS COMMUNICATED

Recovery

- ☐ SAFETY CONCERNS COMMUNICATED
  Airway, Breathing, Circulation (fluid balance), Body Temperature, Pain
- ☐ ASSESSMENT & INTERVENTION PLAN confirmed
- ☐ ANALGESIC PLAN confirmed
- ☐ Person assigned to MONITOR patient

This checklist was written by the AVA with design and distribution support from

Anaesthetic emergencies [2, 10, 18]

Cardiopulmonary resuscitation algorithm

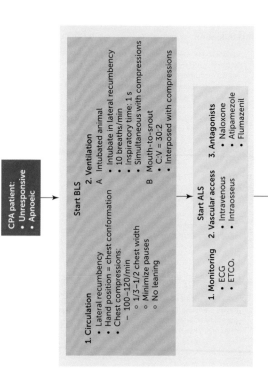

CPA patient:
- Unresponsive
- Apnoeic

Start BLS

1. Circulation
- Lateral recumbency
- Hand position = chest conformation
- Chest compressions:
  - 100–120/min
    - 1/3–1/2 chest width
    - Minimize pauses
    - No leaning

2. Ventilation

A Intubated animal
- Intubate in lateral recumbency
- 10 breaths/min
- Inspiratory time: 1 s
- Simultaneous with compressions

B Mouth-to-snout
- C:V = 30:2
- Interposed with compressions

Start ALS

1. Monitoring
- ECG
- ETCO₂

2. Vascular access
- Intravenous
- Intraosseus

3. Antagonists
- Naloxone
- Atipamezole
- Flumazenil

Basic life support (BLS) is started immediately after recognition of cardiopulmonary arrest (CPA), continued throughout the resuscitation effort and only interrupted every 2 minutes for short patient evaluations (electrocardiogram (ECG) and pulse). Advanced life support (ALS) measures occur whilst BLS is ongoing.

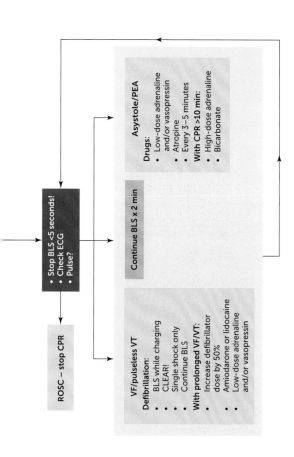

Stop BLS <5 seconds!
- Check ECG
- Pulse?

ROSC – stop CPR

Continue BLS x 2 min

Asystole/PEA

Drugs:
- Low-dose adrenaline and/or vasopressin
- Atropine
- Every 3–5 minutes

With CPR >10 min:
- High-dose adrenaline
- Bicarbonate

VF/pulseless VT

Defibrillation:
- BLS while charging
- CLEAR!
- Single shock only
- Continue BLS

With prolonged VF/VT:
- Increase defibrillator dose by 50%
- Amiodarone or lidocaine
- Low-dose adrenaline and/or vasopressin

C:V = compression:ventilation; ETCO$_2$ = end-tidal carbon dioxide; PEA = pulseless electrical activity; ROSC = return of spontaneous circulation; VF = ventricular fibrillation; VT = ventricular tachycardia.

Contents and use of an anaesthetic emergency box

Drugs

Required:

- Adrenaline (epinephrine)
- Vasopressin
- Atropine
- Lidocaine
- Calcium gluconate
- 50% dextrose
- Isotonic crystalloids (e.g. 0.9% NaCl, lactated Ringer's solution)

May be useful:

- Amiodarone
- Magnesium sulphate
- Furosemide
- Mannitol
- Sodium bicarbonate
- Diazepam/midazolam
- Hypertonic saline
- Naloxone

Equipment

- Pressure bag for rapid fluid infusion
- Manual resuscitator (Ambu) bag
- Endotracheal tubes (various sizes)
- Laryngoscope
- Isopropyl alcohol
- Antiseptic scrub
- Hypodermic needles (various sizes)
- Intravenous catheters (various sizes)
- Gauze sponges/swabs (2 inches x 2 inches (5 x 5 cm), 4 inches x 4 inches (10 x 10 cm))
- Tape (½ inch (1.2 cm), 1 inch (2.5 cm), 2 inches (5 cm))
- Roll of gauze (2 inches (5 cm))
- Polyethylene urinary catheters
- Suture material
- Three-way stopcocks
- Thoracotomy tray with loaded scalpel blade
- Clippers
- Electrocardiogram (ECG) monitor/defibrillator

Crash cart drugs and equipment. (continues) ▶

Equipment *continued*

- Capnograph
- External and sterile internal defibrillator paddles
- Intraosseous cannula placement device and intraosseous cannula
- Airway suctioning device (ready to use)

Other

Emergency drug dosing chart
CPR algorithm poster

(continued) Crash cart drugs and equipment.

NOTES

CPR drug dosing chart

			Weight (kg)	2.5	5	10	15	20	25	30	35	40	45	50
			Weight (lb)	5	10	20	30	40	50	60	70	80	90	100
	Drug	Dose		ml	ml	ml	ml	ml	ml	ml	ml	ml	ml	ml
Arrest	Epi Low (1:1000: 1 mg/ml) every other BLS cycle x3	0.01 mg/kg		0.03	0.05	0.1	0.15	0.2	0.25	0.3	0.35	0.4	0.45	0.5
	Epi High (1:1000: 1 mg/ml) for prolonged CPR	0.1 mg/kg		0.25	0.5	1	1.5	2	2.5	3	3.5	4	4.5	5
	Vasopressin (20 IU/ml)	0.8 IU/kg		0.1	0.2	0.4	0.6	0.8	1	1.2	1.4	1.6	1.8	2
	Atropine (0.54 mg/ml)	0.04 mg/kg		0.2	0.4	0.8	1.1	1.5	1.9	2.2	2.6	3	3.3	3.7
Anti-arrhythmic	Amiodarone (50 mg/ml)	5 mg/kg		0.25	0.5	1	1.5	2	2.5	3	3.5	4	4.5	5
	Lidocaine (20 mg/ml)	2 mg/kg		0.25	0.5	1	1.5	2	2.5	3	3.5	4	4.5	5

Defibrillator dosing is for a monophasic electrical defibrillator.
BLS = basic life support; CPR = cardiopulmonary resuscitation;
Epi = epinephrine (adrenaline). (continues) ▶

	Drug	Dose	Weight (kg) 2.5 / Weight (lb) 5	5 / 10	10 / 20	15 / 30	20 / 40	25 / 50	30 / 60	35 / 70	40 / 80	45 / 90	50 / 100
Reversal	Naloxone (0.4 mg/ml)	0.04 mg/kg	0.25 ml	0.5	1	1.5	2	2.5	3	3.5	4	4.5	5
	Flumazenil (0.1 mg/ml)	0.01 mg/kg	0.25 ml	0.5	1	1.5	2	2.5	3	3.5	4	4.5	5
	Atipamezole (5 mg/ml)	100 µg/kg	0.06 ml	0.1	0.2	0.3	0.4	0.5	0.6	0.7	0.8	0.9	1
Electrical defibrillation	External defib	4–6 J/kg	10	20	40	60	80	100	120	140	160	180	200
	Internal defib	0.5–1 J/kg	2	3	5	8	10	15	15	20	20	20	25

(continued) Defibrillator dosing is for a monophasic electrical defibrillator. BLS = basic life support; CPR = cardiopulmonary resuscitation; Epi = epinephrine (adrenaline).

Anaesthetic equipment [5, 13, 14, 16]

How to choose an anaesthetic breathing circuit

T-piece

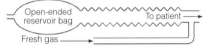

Used for *continuous* IPPV?	Yes
Fresh gas flow rate	500–600 ml/kg/min
Circuit factor	2.5–3
Patient weight range	<10 kg
Can be used with nitrous oxide?	Yes
Advantages	Lightweight, cheap, semi-disposable
Disadvantages	Difficult to scavenge from
Comments	Circuit often now sold with a plastic APL valve and closed reservoir bag that, although not technically a T-piece, can be used in the same way and is easier to scavenge from

Bain

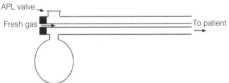

Used for *continuous* IPPV?	Yes
Fresh gas flow rate	400–500 ml/kg/min
Circuit factor	2.5–3

▶

Patient weight range	<15–20 kg
Can be used with nitrous oxide?	Yes
Advantages	Lightweight, cheap, semi-disposable Can be used for continuous IPPV
Disadvantages	High fresh gas flow rates preclude its use in larger animals
Comments	Can be used with a ventilator to provide continuous mechanical IPPV Inner pipe can become disconnected or leak at the anaesthetic machine end, resulting in rebreathing

Lack

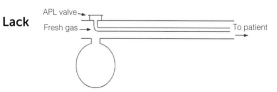

Used for *continuous* IPPV?	No
Fresh gas flow rate	160–200 ml/kg/min
Circuit factor	1–1.5
Patient weight range	>12 kg
Can be used with nitrous oxide?	Yes
Advantages	Lightweight, cheap, semi-disposable Lower flow rates than the Bain
Disadvantages	Not suitable for continuous IPPV
Comments	Inner pipe can become disconnected or leak at the anaesthetic machine end, resulting in rebreathing

Parallel Lack

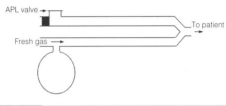

Used for *continuous* IPPV?	No
Fresh gas flow rate	160–200 ml/kg/min
Circuit factor	1–1.5
Patient weight range	>12 kg
Can be used with nitrous oxide?	Yes
Advantages	Lightweight, cheap, semi-disposable Lower flow rates than the Bain
Disadvantages	Parallel breathing pipes increase the drag on the endotracheal tube
Comments	Identical in function to the Lack Leaks or damage more easily identified

Humphrey ADE without soda lime canister

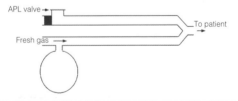

Used for *continuous* IPPV?	Yes
Fresh gas flow rate	100–150 ml/kg/min ▶

Circuit factor	0.5–0.75
Patient weight range	<10 kg
Can be used with nitrous oxide?	Yes
Advantages	Lower flow rates than a standard parallel Lack
Comments	The special APL valve fitted to these circuits maximizes dead-space gas conservation, allowing lower flow rates to be used
The APL valve design might also reduce alveolar collapse during anaesthesia
Suitable for continuous IPPV (and can be configured to work with a mechanical ventilator)

Magill

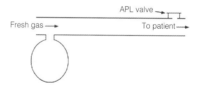

Used for *continuous* IPPV?	No
Fresh gas flow rate	160–200 ml/kg/min
Circuit factor	0.70–1
Patient weight range	>12 kg
Can be used with nitrous oxide?	Yes
Advantages	None
Disadvantages	Valve at the patient end of the circuit is difficult to scavenge
Comments	The Humphrey ADE and parallel Lack have now replaced the Magill and should be preferred

Circle

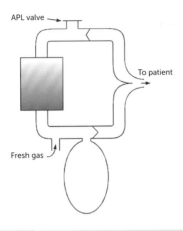

APL valve

To patient

Fresh gas

Used for *continuous* IPPV?	Yes
Fresh gas flow rate	Initially: 2–4 l/min After 5 minutes: 1–2 l/min
Circuit factor	N/A
Patient weight range	>15 kg
Can be used with nitrous oxide?	No, unless respiratory gas monitoring is available
Advantages	Low flow rates reduce costs and environmental pollution
Disadvantages	Large resistance to breathing Not suitable for short procedures
Comments	Do not use with nitrous oxide (unless respiratory gas monitoring is available) The relative positions of the fresh gas inlet, the reservoir bag and the APL valve vary between manufacturers The reservoir bag is best placed on the inspiratory limb. Circle circuits with the inspiratory bag on the expiratory limb offer a much greater resistance to inspiration

Humphrey ADE with soda lime canister

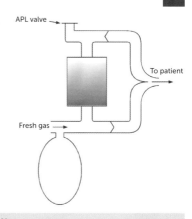

APL valve

To patient

Fresh gas

Used for *continuous* IPPV?	Yes
Fresh gas flow rate	Initially: 30 ml/kg/min After 5 minutes: 10 ml/kg/min (minimum flow 300 ml/min)
Circuit factor	N/A
Patient weight range	>7 kg
Can be used with nitrous oxide?	No, unless respiratory gas monitoring is available
Advantages	Very low flow rates achievable (a 30 kg dog requires only 300 ml/min) reducing costs and environmental pollution Lightweight valves allow it to be used on patients that would not be able to use a normal circle Made of non-ferrous metals so can be used in an MRI scanner The unique APL valve ensures that gas is conserved within the circuit even during rapid respiration
Disadvantages	Initial purchase price is high
Comments	Do not use with nitrous oxide (unless respiratory gas monitoring is available)

The Humphrey ADE circuit

The Humphrey ADE circuit was invented by Dr Humphrey in the 1980s. Because of some of its unique design features, it can be used in animals varying in size from a cat to a Great Dane. The circuit can be used in two basic configurations: with or without soda lime.

Humphrey ADE circuit with soda lime

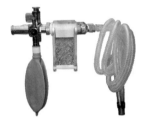

- The Humphrey ADE circuit can be fitted with a soda lime canister, making it into a small circle circuit. This can be used for animals weighing more than 7 kg.

Humphrey ADE circuit without soda lime

- Without soda lime, the circuit works like a Lack with a proportion of the dead-space gas being rebreathed.

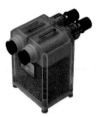

- The narrow smooth-bore tubing means that it can be used on cats, larger birds and reptiles as well as dogs.
- The modified APL valve improves on the efficiency of the normal Lack circuit, allowing lower flow rates than those recommended for a normal Lack circuit to be used safely.

'Lever' on the Humphrey ADE circuit

- The lever on the side of the Humphrey ADE circuit changes its configuration so that it can be used with a mechanical ventilator either with or without the soda lime canister.
- The lever ***must*** be left up, unless the circuit is connected to a ventilator.

The Humphrey APL valve

The Humphrey ADE circuit is fitted with a special APL valve that contributes to the circuit's efficiency. Like a parallel Lack, it is possible to reduce the fresh gas flow used until the animal starts to rebreathe the dead-space gas from the previous breath. Of the gas exhaled by an animal, 30–40% is dead-space gas and, as it is free of carbon dioxide, it can be conserved in the breathing circuit and delivered to the patient during the next breath. In theory, the exhaled dead-space gases in a Lack and parallel Lack pass back down the inspiratory limb of the circuit until the reservoir bag is full. Then the alveolar gases pass down the expiratory limb towards the APL valve. In practice, the APL valve opens before the reservoir bag is full and some of the dead-space gas is lost.

The Humphrey APL valve is designed not to open until the reservoir bag is full, conserving more of the dead-space gas in the inspiratory limb of the circuit.

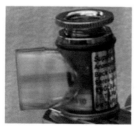
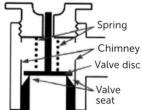

Spring

Chimney

Valve disc

Valve seat

The Humphrey APL valve has another benefit. During anaesthesia, the alveoli in the dependent (lower) lung lobes collapse and do not fill with anaesthetic gases. This reduces gas exchange and can contribute to hypoxia in patients with compromised pulmonary function. The APL valve on the Humphrey ADE circuit closes earlier in the breathing cycle, maintaining a slight positive pressure (1 cmH$_2$O) in the circuit and the patient's lungs. In children this has been demonstrated to prevent alveolar collapse and it is likely that the same benefit exists in small animals.

Phase 1 – Early expiration

The pressure in the circuit rises and the valve disc lifts off the valve seat, but the valve effectively remains closed as the valve disc does not get pushed completely out of the valve chimney. This prevents the dead-space gas from leaving the circuit and it must all flow into the *inspiratory* limb, where it is conserved.

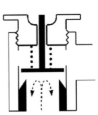

Phase 2 – Late expiration

Once the reservoir bag is full the pressure in the circuit rises still further, lifting the valve disc beyond the valve chimney and allowing the alveolar gases to escape into the scavenging system.

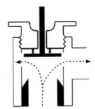

Phase 3 – Expiratory pause

At the end of expiration the valve closes again but the valve disc falls back into the chimney at a pressure of 1 cmH$_2$O, preventing the last few millilitres of gas from escaping and maintaining a slight positive pressure in the circuit *and* in the patient's lungs during the expiratory pause. In children at least, this prevents alveolar collapse.

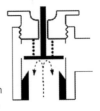

Phase 4 – Inspiration

The valve disc is held against the valve seat by the spring, preventing gas from being drawn back in from the atmosphere. This prevents carbon dioxide-rich alveolar gas now sitting in the expiratory limb from being drawn back towards the patient. The patient must breathe carbon dioxide-free dead-space gas and fresh gas from the inspiratory limb.

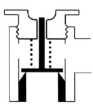

Calculating fresh gas flow rates

Due to the reliance on the fresh gas flow rate to prevent rebreathing in systems without a soda lime canister, correct calculation of fresh gas flow rate is essential.

1. Calculate the patient's **tidal volume** (TV). This is the volume of gas exhaled in one breath and is considered to be between 10 and 15 ml/kg.

    *   The size of the patient is the first thing to consider when determining which end of the 10–15 ml/kg range to use. Generally, use the high end of the range for small dogs and cats. For larger patients, e.g. Labradors, a tidal volume of 10 ml/kg is appropriate.
    *   Consider the body condition of the patient. Only the lean weight, i.e. what the bodyweight would be at a body condition score of 3/5, should be used in the calculation.
    *   Consider the shape of the patient's thorax. Deep-chested breeds such as Greyhounds will have a higher tidal volume than would be expected for their bodyweight (12–15 ml/kg).

        Tidal volume (ml) = **10–15 × bodyweight** (kg)

▪▪▶

2. Calculate the patient's **minute volume** (MV). This is the volume of gas expired by the patient in 1 minute and requires measurement of respiratory rate (breaths per minute). This should be done when the patient has been allowed to acclimatize to its environment. The best way of gathering this information is to observe the patient from a distance when it is in its kennel. If the patient is panting, the respiratory rate should be estimated. Once the patient is anaesthetized the respiratory rate may be different to that used for the MV calculation. It is important to recalculate MV if the respiratory rate increases, as it will lead to increased MV.

> **Minute volume** (ml/min) =
> **Tidal volume** (ml) × **Respiratory rate** (/min)

3. Multiply the calculated minute volume by the **circuit factor** of the breathing system being used. The circuit factor varies between different breathing systems.

> **Fresh gas flow rate** (ml/min) =
> **Minute volume** (ml/min) × **Circuit factor**

EXAMPLE 1
DSH cat, 4.5 kg, respiratory rate 32 breaths/min

Tidal volume	= 4.5 x 15 = 67.5 ml
Minute volume	= 67.5 x 32 = 2160 ml

T-piece circuit selected (low resistance, low dead space, low TV).

Fresh gas flow rate = MV x circuit factor = 2160 x 2.5
= 5400 ml (5.4 litres)

The veterinary surgeon requests that nitrous oxide is used.

O_2 flow rate	= 5400 ÷ 3 = 1800 ml (c.2 litres)
N_2O flow rate	= 1800 x 2 = 3600 ml (c.3.5 litres)

▶

EXAMPLE 1 *continued*

Once the cat is anaesthetized its respiratory rate reduces to 16 breaths/min, allowing recalculation of flow rate. This is not absolutely necessary and maintaining a high flow rate will do no harm, but will increase costs and increase environmental contamination.

Minute volume = 67.5 x 16 = 1080 ml

Fresh gas flow rate
= 1080 x 2.5 = 2700 ml
$\qquad$ (3 litres – 1 litre of O_2 + 2 litres of N_2O)

EXAMPLE 2

Labrador, 25 kg, respiratory rate 16 breaths/min

Tidal volume	= 25 x 10 = 250 ml
Minute volume	= 250 x 16 = 4000 ml

Lack selected (lower requirement for fresh gas flow compared to a Bain, ease of circuit use compared to a Magill).

Fresh gas flow rate = MV x circuit factor
$\qquad$ = 4000 x 1 = 4000 ml (4 litres)

A circle system could also be used in a semi-closed configuration. This could be achieved by using a fresh gas flow rate of 3 litres/min for the first 20 minutes to ensure denitrogenation and then reducing the fresh gas flow rate to 1 litre/min.

NOTES

Checking anaesthetic equipment

Checking the anaesthetic machine

A check should be performed at the start of each day before the anaesthetic machine is used. The following steps comprise a check of anaesthetic machine function:

1. Attach the scavenging pipe to the appropriate exhaust port and switch on the active scavenging system (if available).
2. Perform a visual check of the anaesthetic machine and associated pipelines and cylinders; ensure cylinders are seated within the yoke correctly and firmly.
3. Open cylinders and check content; change if necessary.
4. Turn on O_2 flow; check the bobbin moves slowly from low to high flows with the bobbin/ball spinning continuously. Turn the flow to 4 l/min. Repeat for N_2O if present.
5. Turn off O_2 cylinder and press oxygen flush; as the flow drops, the O_2 supply failure alarm will sound and N_2O should cut off (if a hypoxic guard is present on machine).
6. If an O_2 pipeline is available, connect. If not, switch the O_2 cylinder on. Flow should resume to 4 l/min.
7. Check pipeline pressure (most run at around 4.2 bar). Press O_2 flush; the pressure should only drop slightly (contact engineer if the drop is greater than 0.5 bar).
8. Switch off N_2O.
9. With the O_2 flow at 4 l/min, occlude the common gas outlet with your thumb; watch that the bobbin drops and listen for the pressure relief valve to open (sounds like a small hiss/squeak); release the occlusion (not all anaesthetic machines have a pressure relief valve on the back bar).

Checking the vaporizer

The vaporizer should be checked at the start of each day before use:

1. Check vaporizer content (vaporizers should be filled at end of the day to reduce exposure to personnel); if using the selectatec system, ensure that the vaporizer is seated on the back bar correctly and locked into place.
2. Check the dial rotates smoothly.
3. With the vaporizer switched on but set to zero, occlude the common gas outlet with your thumb; ensure that the bobbin drops (release pressure as soon as a drop is observed). This is performed to check there is no leak present on the interface between the anaesthetic machine and vaporizer.

Checking breathing systems

Breathing systems should be checked before every use. The basic principle is the same whatever the breathing system, with small variations towards the end of the check to test individual special features. The following checks should be performed on all breathing systems:

1. Visually check for any contamination (e.g. blood) or obvious damage/holes in the tubing or reservoir bag. Dispose of damaged circuits or clean if necessary. Individual parts can often be replaced without the need to replace the whole circuit.
2. Check that the components of the system are in the correct location, e.g. the valve and reservoir bag.
3. Attach the gas inlet on the breathing system to the common gas outlet of the anaesthetic machine and attach the scavenging system.
4. Close the APL valve or, in the case of the Jackson–Rees modified Ayres T-piece, occlude the neck of the bag where it enters the scavenging system.
5. Occlude the patient attachment end, either with your hand or hold it against your leg (whichever method it is important to create an airtight seal). ▪▶

6. Fill the system with O_2 (or medical air if available). This can be done either by using the oxygen flush or the flowmeters. Stop gas flow once the reservoir bag is distended.
7. Listen and feel for any leaks.
8. Open the APL valve and squeeze the contents out of the reservoir bag to check that the valve opens fully. It is important whilst doing this to keep the patient attachment occluded.

Additional checks should be carried out for coaxial systems, to confirm that there is no damage to the inner limb.

- **Bain:** With the O_2 flowmeter set at 4 litres and the valve closed, use a pen (or disposable Bain breathing systems come with a plastic tool of the correct diameter) to occlude the inner limb. Observe the bobbin within the flowmeter – it will dip if there are no leaks in the system. It should only be transiently occluded as it causes back pressure within the anaesthetic machine, which could be damaging.
- **Lack:** With the O_2 flowmeter set at 4 litres and the valve closed, use a pen of a similar diameter (or disposable Lacks come with a plastic tool of the correct diameter) to occlude the inner limb. Observe the reservoir bag filling and becoming distended.

NOTES

ASA physical status and classifications scale[5]

ASA scale	Physical description	Veterinary patient examples
1	Normal patient with no disease	Healthy patient scheduled for ovariohysterectomy or castration
2	Patient with mild systemic disease that does not limit normal function	Controlled diabetes mellitus, mild cardiac valve insufficiency
3	Patient with moderate systemic disease that limits normal function	Uncontrolled diabetes mellitus, symptomatic heart disease
4	Patient with severe systemic disease that is a constant threat to life	Sepsis, organ failure, heart failure
5	Patient that is moribund and not expected to live 24 hours without surgery	Shock, multiple organ failure, severe trauma
E	Describes patient as an emergency	Gastric dilatation–volvulus, respiratory distress

NOTES

Bandaging [13, 16]

Foot and lower limb bandage

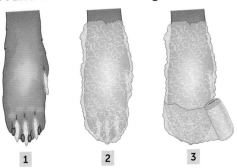

1. Cut long claws. Pad out the toes using a small piece of absorbent dressing.
2. Apply a padding layer over the foot covering the dorsal and palmar/plantar area.
3. Twist the bandage to cover diagonally the medial and lateral aspect of the foot.

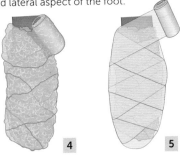

4. Roll the bandage in a proximal direction spiralling up the leg to cover the joint above the area to be bandaged.
5. Repeat this for the conforming layer and the cohesive layer.

Ear and head bandage

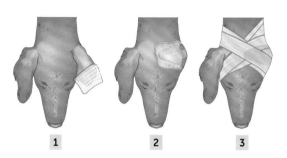

1. Cover any wounds with an appropriate sterile dressing.
2. Place padding on top of cranium. Pick up ear by tip of pinna and lay flat back on padding; repeat if including both ears. Place padding on top of pinna.
3. Place padding under neck. Wrap conforming layer in a figure-of-eight pattern until the area is covered, using the free ear for additional anchorage.

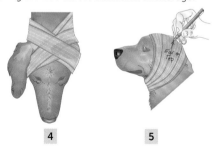

4. Cover the bandage with a cohesive layer following a similar pattern.
5. Use marker pen to indicate on the outer layer the position of the pinna. Make sure that the bandage does not interfere with swallowing or breathing. ▪▪➡

Thoracic bandage

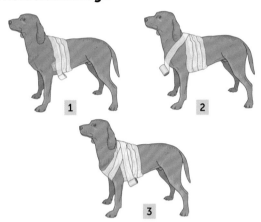

1. Apply a sterile dressing to any wounds. Starting dorsally mid thorax apply a padding layer around the chest wall.
2. Incorporate the forelimbs in a figure-of-eight to help secure the bandage.
3. Return along the chest wall, ending caudally to where the bandage started.

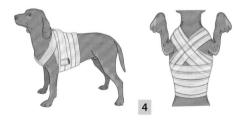

4. Cover the padded layer with a conforming bandage. Make sure that the bandage is not too tight and does not compromise respiratory efforts.

Abdominal bandage

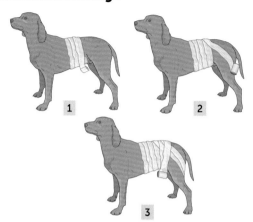

1. Apply a sterile dressing to any wounds. Starting mid abdomen, apply a padding layer around the abdominal wall.
2. Incorporate the hindlimbs in a figure-of-eight to help secure the bandage.
3. Return along the abdominal wall, ending cranially to where the bandage started.

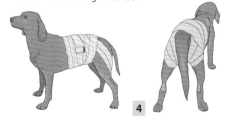

4. Cover the padded layer with a conforming bandage. Pay particular attention to anatomy of genitalia in both male and female animals – be careful not to cover prepuce or vulva.

Tail bandage

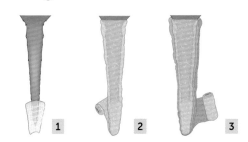

1. Use an appropriate dressing to cover the wound.
2. Using a conforming bandage, roll from the base, along the dorsal aspect of the tail, to the tip of the tail. Go under the tip, along the ventral aspect of the tail and back to the base.
3. Fold the bandage back on itself and return along the ventral surface to the tip of the tail.

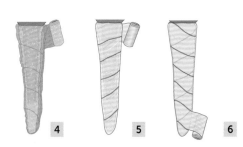

4. Spiral the bandage from the tip in a proximal direction towards the base, ensuring even pressure up to the base of the tail.
5. Apply a cohesive layer using the same methodology; from tip to base.
6. Return from base to tip.

Ehmer sling

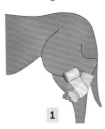

1

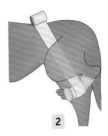

2

1. Lightly pad the metatarsal area (this prevents swelling, though too much padding will cause the bandage to slip). Secure conforming bandage around the metatarsal area from the medial to the lateral aspect.
2. Flex the whole limb, turning the foot inwards (this will turn the hock outwards and the stifle inwards, immobilizing the hip). Bring the bandage up under the medial aspect of the stifle. A small amount of padding may be applied to the cranial aspect of the stifle.

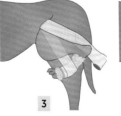

3

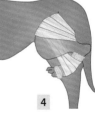

4

3. Bring the bandage over the lateral aspect of the thigh and around the medial aspect of the hock, returning to the lateral aspect of the metatarsals.
4. Apply several more layers until the leg is secure and the hip is supported. Repeat this for the cohesive dressing as required. Tension of the bandage must be checked carefully on application: if too tight, it could result in ischaemic damage to the lower limb. ⅢⅢ➡

Velpeau sling

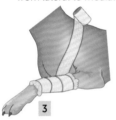

1. Pad the carpal area.
2. Secure conforming bandage over the carpal area, from lateral to medial.

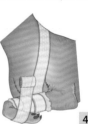
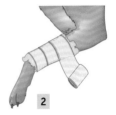

3. Bring the bandage from the medial carpus, up over the lateral aspect of the shoulder and around the opposite side of the chest behind the contralateral elbow.
4. Ensure the carpus, elbow and shoulder are flexed, and incorporate the carpus into the sling.
5. Repeat this until the complete forelimb has been covered, producing a sling effect. The whole bandage can be covered with a cohesive layer. Tension of the bandage must be checked carefully on application: if too tight it could result in ischaemic damage to the lower limb.

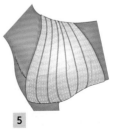

Robert Jones bandage

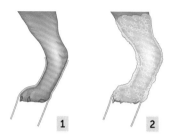

1. Place two lengths of zinc oxide tape to cover 15–20 cm up the leg and 10–13 cm overlap at the toes and place on each side of the leg to form stirrups. Pad out toes as necessary.
2. Place cotton wool layer: start halfway up nail and reverse roll cotton wool four or five times around the leg.

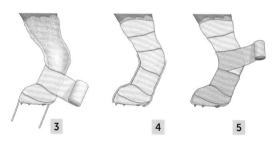

3. Place conforming bandage: this should compress the cotton wool as firmly and as evenly as possible and should cover it entirely.
4. Unstick the two ends of zinc oxide tape and fold back to secure the bandage.
5. Cover the bandage with cohesive dressing.

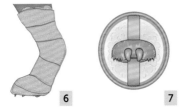

6. Check that the bandage is not too tight: it should be possible to insert two fingers between the bandage and the animal. When flicked, the bandage should sound like a ripe melon.
7. The two middle toes should remain exposed.

See also **Wound dressings** *and* **Wound drain management**

NOTES

Biochemistry reference ranges [16]

Biochemical parameter	Dogs	Cats
Albumin (g/l)	25–40	25–40
Alanine aminotransferase (ALT) (IU/l)	10–75	35–134
Alkaline phosphatase (ALP) (IU/l)	0–80	15–96
Blood urea nitrogen (mmol/l)	2.5–7	5–11
Calcium (mmol/l)	2–3	1.8–3
Cholesterol (mmol/l)	2.5–8	2–6.5
Creatinine (µmol/l)	40–130	40–130
Glucose (mmol/l)	3.3–6	3.3–6
Pancreatic amylase (IU/l)	350–1200	515–2210
Phosphate (mmol/l)	0.8–1.6	1.3–2.6
Total bilirubin (µmol/l)	1.7–10	2–5
Total protein (g/l)	54–71	54–78

NB: Reference ranges will vary with laboratory; these are averages

See also **Haematology reference ranges**

Biosecurity *see* **Infection control**

Blood cell types [16]

Cell type	Normal appearance	Description	Role/significance
Erythrocyte		Pink, biconcave disc with no nucleus	Transport of blood gases
Mature neutrophil		Multi-lobed nucleus, pale granules in cytoplasm	Phagocytosis
Immature neutrophil		Horseshoe-shaped nucleus	Phagocytosis
Eosinophil		Pink granules with bilobed or segmented nucleus	Increased in parasitic conditions
Basophil		Irregular nucleus with blue granular cytoplasm	Increased in allergic reactions
Lymphocyte		Larger cells, nucleus occupies majority of cell	Immune response: B cells and T cells
Monocyte		Horse-shaped nucleus. Larger cells. No granules in cytoplasm	Phagocytosis
Thrombocyte		Very small cells	Clotting

(Courtesy of Axiom Laboratories)

NOTES

Blood collection tubes [2, 16]

EDTA (ethylene diamine tetra-acetic acid)	
Universal *	Pink
Vacutainer *	Mauve
Sample	Whole blood
Tests	Haematology
Comments	Fill tube precisely to level indicated. Underfilling may cause artefacts; overfilling may lead to clotting
None	
Universal *	White Brown
Vacutainer *	Red
Sample	Serum
Tests	Biochemistry; bile acids; serology
Serum gel	
Universal *	Brown
Vacutainer *	Gold
Sample	Serum
Tests	Biochemistry; bile acids; serology
Lithium heparin	
Universal *	Orange
Vacutainer *	Green
Sample	Plasma
Tests	Biochemistry; electrolytes
Comments	Do not use blood that has been mixed with EDTA
Sodium fluoride and potassium oxalate	
Universal *	Yellow
Vacutainer *	Grey

*Always check cap colour codes, as they may vary with manufacturer. (continues) ▶

Sodium fluoride and potassium oxalate continued	
Sample	Whole blood
Tests	Blood glucose
Comments	Fluoride/oxalate inhibits red blood cells oxidizing glucose
Sodium citrate	
Universal *	Blue
Vacutainer *	Blue
Sample	Whole blood
Tests	Coagulation tests; platelet counts

(continued) *Always check cap colour codes, as they may vary with manufacturer.

NOTES

Blood pressure measurement [2]

Direct blood pressure measurement

Invasive blood pressure measurement by means of an arterial catheter is considered the 'gold standard' technique but is technically demanding in terms of placement of the catheter, maintaining patency of the arterial catheter and ensuring accurate 'zeroing' of the apparatus to ambient air at the level of the right atrium.

Indications/Use

- Monitoring arterial blood pressure in critically ill patients.
- Monitoring arterial blood pressure during anaesthesia.
- Arterial catheters can also be used for serial collection of arterial blood samples for blood gas analysis in animals with pulmonary disease.

Contraindications

- Coagulopathy.
- Arterial catheters should not be placed at sites where risk of bacterial contamination and infection are high, e.g. due to local tissue damage, local skin infection, diarrhoea, urinary incontinence.

Equipment

- No. 11 scalpel.
- 20–22 G peripheral venous over-the-needle catheter.
- T-connector or extension set containing heparinized saline (1 IU of heparin per ml of 0.9% saline).
- 70% surgical spirit.
- Adhesive tape.
- Soft padded bandage and outer protective bandage.
- Non-compliant manometer tubing.
- Pressure transducer: must be 'zeroed' to ambient air at the level of the right atrium.
- Display monitor.
- Pressurized continuous flush system.

Patient preparation and positioning

- The patient should be positioned in lateral recumbency.
- The patient's limb must be held still; this can be achieved by manual restraint.
- For monitoring of the anaesthetized patient, arterial catheters should be placed soon after anaesthetic induction, and before the animal's blood pressure falls, as low BP makes palpation of a peripheral arterial pulse more challenging.

Sites

- The dorsal pedal artery in the hindpaw is most commonly used.
- Other arteries that may be used include: the femoral artery; auricular artery; and palmar metacarpal artery in the forepaw.

The dorsal pedal artery

Technique

1. Place a catheter into a peripheral artery:
   - Palpate the arterial pulse
   - The skin overlying the artery is clipped, then sprayed or lightly wiped with surgical spirit. Excessive scrubbing/wiping of the skin should be avoided, as this may result in spasm of the artery
   - Make a small stab incision in the skin overlying the arterial pulse
   - A peripheral venous catheter is placed through the skin incision and then inserted into the artery using short, firm, purposeful movements to push the stylet and catheter through the muscular wall of the artery. For entry into the artery, the catheter should be positioned at a slight angle to the artery – approximately 10–30 degrees
   - The dorsal pedal artery runs at about 30 degrees to the long axis of the metatarsus from medial to lateral. During catheter placement, palpate ➠

the arterial pulse constantly, proximal to the site of entry of the catheter into the artery. This allows the operator to guide the catheter tip towards the artery, which cannot be seen

- As soon as arterial blood is seen in the flash chamber of the catheter, the stylet and catheter are lowered to a position parallel to the artery and advanced together a little further into the artery, before the catheter is advanced over the stylet and completely into the artery
- Withdraw the catheter stylet and attach a T-connector or extension set containing heparinized saline to the catheter. Arterial blood should be seen to pulsate within the hub of the catheter or T-connector
- The catheter should be secured firmly in place with adhesive tape and covered with a bandage.

The bandage over an arterial catheter must be labelled clearly to avoid inadvertent administration of fluids or drugs into an artery.

2. Connect the T-connector to a pressure transducer via non-compliant tubing filled with heparinized saline.
3. To allow trouble-free continuous monitoring (avoiding clotting in the arterial line), the set-up is combined with a pressurized continuous flush system. If this is not available, arterial catheters should be flushed hourly.
4. The transducer–monitor combination gives a continuous reading of blood pressure and shows the pressure waveform. Systolic and diastolic pressures are taken as the cyclic maximum and minimum pressures, respectively. Mean pressure is calculated automatically. Arterial blood pressure monitoring is usually continuous.

5. On removal of the catheter, apply direct pressure to the artery for 5 minutes, then wrap with a light pressure dressing, e.g. folded gauze swab secured in place over the artery with adhesive tape.

Potential complications

■ Excessive arterial bleeding/exsanguination following a failed attempt at catheterization or accidental removal of the catheter.
■ Vascular damage and subsequent tissue necrosis distal to the catheter. The risk of this complication can be minimized by:
  - Avoiding placing adhesive tape too tightly around the paw
  - Never using arterial catheters for giving drugs or fluids
  - Regular monitoring of the catheter and paw; arterial catheters should be checked every hour
  - Prompt removal of arterial catheters when they are no longer required.
■ Infection.
■ Thrombosis/thromboembolism.
■ Embolism of a piece of catheter due to accidental transection of the catheter with a blade or scissors.
■ Air embolism.

NOTES

Indirect blood pressure measurement

Non-invasive blood pressure measurements are technically less demanding than invasive measurements and can be rapidly applied in the emergency situation, although they might not fulfil the expectations of reliability and accuracy. There are two non-invasive methods in general use: the oscillometric method and the Doppler method. Both require a cuff.

Indications/Use
- To assess cardiovascular function.
- Routine monitoring during anaesthesia.

Equipment
- Doppler ultrasound probe.
- Coupling gel.
- Adhesive tape.
- Inflatable cuff attached to a manometer.

OR
- Oscillometric blood pressure monitor with cuffs.

CUFF SIZE

The proper cuff width is 40% of the circumference of the site where the cuff will be placed. Cuffs that are too wide lead to falsely low readings; those that are too narrow lead to falsely high readings.

Patient preparation and positioning
- Can be performed on conscious, sedated or anaesthetized animals.
  - **NB:** Assessment of general cardiovascular status should be made in the absence of sedative and anaesthetic drugs.
- For conscious animals, it is important that they are relaxed. A quiet, stress-free environment is ideal. Allow the animal a period of at least 5–10 minutes to relax.

- The limb used should not be weight-bearing and the animal should be positioned such that the cuff is at the level of the right atrium.
- For the Doppler technique, it is necessary to prepare the skin overlying the artery to be used for blood pressure measurement. Normally the fur should be removed by shaving. However, in cats with short fur, wiping down the fur with surgical spirit may be adequate. Common sites for the detection of an arterial pulse using the Doppler technique are:
  - The palmar arterial arch, on the ventral aspect of the proximal metacarpal region
  - The plantar arterial arch, on the ventral aspect of the proximal metatarsal region
  - The median caudal artery on the ventral aspect of the tail.

Technique

Doppler ultrasound

An inflatable cuff attached to a manometer occludes an artery, and a piezoelectric crystal placed over the artery distal to the cuff detects flow. The re-entry of blood into the artery as the cuff is released causes a frequency change (Doppler shift) in the sound waves. This is detected by the piezoelectric crystal and converted to a sound that is detected by the operator. **This method primarily measures systolic pressure. Recordings of diastolic pressures may be inaccurate.**

1. Apply coupling gel directly to the transducer with the machine switched off.
2. Turn the machine on. Gently position the Doppler ultrasound probe over the prepared skin. Listen carefully for a pulse signal, moving the probe gently until a clear signal can be heard. Secure the probe to the prepared area with adhesive tape.
3. If no signal is heard, consider:
   - Applying more coupling gel

- Securing the probe to the prepared skin before hearing a signal. Excessive digital pressure on the probe may occlude the artery, whereas the pressure from the tape alone may be less, allowing the pulse signal to be heard.

4. Attach the cuff to a handheld sphygmomanometer. Place the cuff around the limb or tail proximal to the probe, avoiding the joints. In dogs, the cuff should be applied snugly enough to allow insertion of only a small finger between the cuff and the leg or tail. Most cuffs have a mark that should be placed directly over the artery.

PRACTICAL TIP

If the cuff is applied too tightly, the measurement will be erroneously low because the cuff partly occludes the artery; if applied too loosely, the measurement will be erroneously high because greater cuff pressure will be required to occlude the artery.

---

5. Gently inflate the cuff using the sphygmomanometer. Inflate the cuff an additional 10–20 mmHg beyond the point at which the pulse can no longer be heard.

6. Slowly deflate the cuff and listen carefully for a return of the pulse signal. The systolic blood pressure reading is the pressure at which the pulse can first be clearly heard.

7. Continue deflating the cuff and listen for the point (diastolic pressure) at which the audio signal of the pulse returns to pre-inflation quality. Thereafter completely deflate the cuff.

8. In a conscious animal, 6–8 blood pressure measurements should be taken to ensure reliability. Discard the first measurement if it is very different from the others. Variability in systolic readings should be <20%. Record the mean systolic and diastolic pressures.

Oscillometric technique

This uses a cuff to occlude the artery, and detects oscillations of the underlying artery when it is partly occluded. **This system determines systolic, diastolic and mean arterial pressures.** This method is less accurate in very small patients, patients with low blood pressure and patients with dysrhythmias. Muscle contractions also create oscillations and are a source of potential error.

1. Place the cuff snugly (see Step 4 above) over one of the following:
   - The radial artery proximal to the carpus
   - The saphenous artery proximal to the tarsus
   - The brachial artery proximal to the elbow
   - The median caudal artery at the base of the tail.
2. Attach the cuff to a control unit that continually senses arterial pressure and inflates to a pressure greater than the systolic, and then automatically deflates the cuff.
3. The heart rate is displayed. Verify that this matches the patient's heart rate by manually counting the rate using direct heart auscultation or palpation of an artery.
4. Record the values for 3–5 cycles and report the averages for systolic, diastolic and mean pressures.

Potential false readings

Incorrect blood pressure readings may be obtained due to:

- Inappropriate cuff size
- Inappropriate placement of the cuff
- Excessive motion of the limb or tail
- Low blood pressure
- Dysrhythmias
- Obesity
- Peripheral oedema
- Limb conformation that does not permit snug placement of the cuff
- Stress.

Blood pressure values for dogs and cats [6, 10]

Blood pressure classification	Systolic BP (mmHg)	Diastolic BP (mmHg)
Hypotension	<90	<50
Normal	Dog: 110–190 Cat: 120–170	Dog: 55–100 Cat: 70–120
Minimal risk of hypertensive TOD	<150	<95
Mild risk of hypertensive TOD	150–159	95–99
Moderate risk of hypertensive TOD	160–179	100–119
Severe risk of hypertensive TOD	>180	>120

TOD = target organ damage

NOTES

Blood sampling [2, 16]

Arterial blood sampling

Indications/Use
- To obtain a sample of arterial blood for assessment of:
  - Respiratory function
  - Arterial oxygen concentration
  - Acid–base status.

Contraindications
- Severe coagulopathy.
- Sampling should not be performed at sites where the risk of bacterial contamination and infection is high, e.g. due to local tissue damage, local skin infection, diarrhoea, urinary incontinence.

Equipment
- A pre-heparinized arterial blood gas syringe with a 23–25 G, $5/8$ inch needle attached.
- 70% surgical spirit.
- Cotton wool or gauze swabs.
- 25 mm wide cohesive bandage (e.g. Vetrap).

Patient preparation and positioning
- Arterial blood sampling is performed in the conscious animal.
- Sedation should be avoided if possible as it will affect test results.
- Animals should be positioned appropriately for the blood collection site (see below).

Sites
Most commonly the dorsal pedal artery is used, but in cats and small dogs it is sometimes easier to use the femoral artery.

Dorsal pedal artery

- The animal is placed in lateral recumbency, either on a table (cats and small dogs) or on the floor (large dogs), with the leg to be sampled placed closest to the table or floor.
- An assistant restrains the patient's head with one hand and the uppermost hindlimb with the other.
- The artery is palpated just distal to the tarsus (hock), between the second and third metatarsal bones, on the dorsal aspect.

Femoral artery

- The animal is placed in lateral recumbency, either on a table (cats and small dogs) or on the floor (large dogs), with the leg to be sampled placed closest to the table or floor.
- The animal is restrained manually, and the upper limb abducted so that the femoral artery can be palpated.
- The femoral artery pulse is palpable on the medial thigh, ventral to the inguinal region and proximal to the stifle.

Technique

1. Stretch the skin over the artery.
2. Palpate the artery.
3. The skin overlying the artery is gently clipped, then sprayed or lightly wiped with surgical spirit. Excessive scrubbing/wiping of the skin should be avoided, as this may result in spasm of the artery.
4. Gently rest two fingertips of one hand against the artery, so that the arterial pulse can be felt.
5. With the other hand, direct the needle, with the syringe attached, towards the artery, at an angle of about 30 degrees. The needle bevel is pointed upwards.

6. Penetrate the artery in one quick firm purposeful movement.
7. When the artery has been penetrated, a flash of blood will be seen in the hub of the needle.
8. Collect approximately 1 ml of blood.
9. Remove the syringe and needle from the artery.
10. On removal of the needle, apply direct pressure to the artery for 5 minutes, then cover with cotton wool or a gauze swab and cohesive bandage.
11. Hold the syringe upright and tap it to cause air bubbles to rise. Eject any air from the syringe.
12. Cap the sample with an airtight seal to prevent exposure to room air. Rubber bungs or plastic caps are available with pre-heparinized blood gas syringes.
13. The blood sample must be analysed as soon as possible, **ideally within 5 minutes.**

Parameter	Dogs	Cats
pH	7.35–7.46	7.31–7.46
PCO_2	30.8–42.8 mmHg (4.10–5.69 kPa)	25.2–36.8 mmHg (3.35–4.89 kPa)
PO_2	80.9–103.3 mmHg (10.76–13.74 kPa)	95.4–118.2 mmHg (12.69–15.72 kPa)
$[HCO_3^-]$	18.8–25.6 mmol/l	14.4–21.6 mmol/l
Base excess	0 ± 4	0 ± 4

Approximate normal arterial blood gas values for dogs and cats breathing room air.

Potential complications

- Significant haemorrhage is very uncommon, provided direct pressure is applied to the artery (see above).
- Bruising and the formation of a small haematoma will occur in some patients, but can be minimized by good technique and by the application of direct pressure to the artery.
- Arterial thrombosis and thrombophlebitis are uncommon, but are more likely if repeated attempts are made to collect blood from an artery. ▸▸▸

Venous blood sampling

Indications/Use

- To obtain a sample of venous blood for clinical pathology tests or for bacterial culture.

Contraindications

- Coagulopathy.
- Sampling should not be performed at sites where risk of bacterial contamination and infection are high, e.g. due to local tissue damage, local skin infection, diarrhoea, urinary incontinence.

Equipment

- Hypodermic needles:
  - Cats: 23–21 G; $^5/_8$ inch
  - Dogs: 21 G; $^5/_8$ or 1 inch.
- 2–10 ml syringes.
- 70% surgical spirit.
- 4% chlorhexidine gluconate or 10% povidone–iodine.
- Cotton wool or gauze swabs.
- 25 mm wide cohesive bandage (e.g. Vetrap).
- Appropriate blood containers (*see* **Blood collection tubes**) and/or three blood culture bottles (pre-warmed to 37°C).
- Sterile gloves.

Patient preparation and positioning

- Venous blood sampling is performed in the conscious animal, although in fractious animals light sedation may be required.
- Cats can be wrapped in a large towel to control their limbs when sampling from the jugular vein; for sampling a peripheral vein the target limb can be excluded from the towel.
- The animal should be positioned appropriately for the blood collection site (see below).

- A generous area over the target vein should be clipped, sufficient to allow identification of the vein, and of the direction in which it runs.
- Using cotton wool or gauze swabs, clean the skin over the vein with 4% chlorhexidine or 10% povidone–iodine, followed by spraying or wiping with surgical spirit.
- When taking samples for bacterial culture, take care not to touch the site of needle insertion. If necessary, gloves should be worn.

Sites

The jugular vein is usually preferred, as it is large enough to allow a sample to be withdrawn rapidly without requiring excessive negative pressure. This minimizes haemolysis and blood clot formation within the sample. The cephalic vein and the lateral saphenous vein may be used: if the jugular vein is not accessible; if the animal resents being restrained for jugular sampling; or if there is a planned procedure that may be compromised by jugular vein haematoma or haemorrhage (e.g. jugular catheter placement or thyroid surgery).

Jugular vein

- The animal is placed in a sitting position, either on a table (cats and small dogs) or on the floor (large dogs).
- An assistant stands on the left of the patient.
- The assistant places their right arm over the patient's back and round the front of the patient, to encircle and control the forelimbs.
- The assistant's left arm is used to extend the animal's neck by grasping its muzzle and directing the nostrils towards the ceiling.
- Fear-aggressive cats, or those that are especially wriggly, can be restrained for jugular sampling by

placing them on their side or on their back,
controlling the limbs with the hands and body, or
wrapping the cat in a towel.
- Raise the vein with one hand by applying gentle
  pressure to the jugular groove at around the level of
  the jugular inlet.

Cephalic vein

- The animal is placed in a sitting position or
  in sternal recumbency, either on a table (cats and
  small dogs) or on the floor (large dogs).
- An assistant stands on the left of the patient.
- The assistant passes their left hand under the patient's
  neck and holds the head turned away from the
  sampler.
- The assistant's right arm is used to extend the patient's
  right forelimb.
- The assistant holding the animal raises the vein by
  wrapping a thumb around the forelimb just distal to
  the elbow, and then gently rotating their wrist to
  encourage the vein on to the cranial aspect of the
  forelimb.

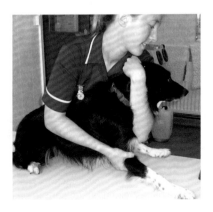

Lateral saphenous vein

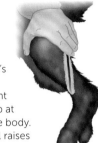

- The animal is placed in lateral recumbency, either on a table (cats and small dogs) or on the floor (large dogs).
- An assistant restrains the animal's head with one hand.
- With the other hand, the assistant extends the uppermost hindlimb at the same time stretching out the body.
- The assistant holding the animal raises the vein by encircling the caudal aspect of the upper hindlimb, applying pressure at the level of the stifle.

Technique

For biochemical tests or haematology

1. Insert the needle into the vein, with syringe attached and the bevel upwards, at an angle of approximately 30 degrees.
2. Follow the line of the vein with the needle tip.
3. Aspirate blood by applying gentle negative pressure to the syringe plunger. Avoid excessive suction on the syringe, as this may collapse the vein. If no blood is present in the hub, try gently redirecting the needle to enter the vein, but avoid large sweeping movements. If necessary, withdraw the needle and start again with a fresh one.
4. Release the pressure on the vein.
5. Remove the needle. If sampling was from the jugular vein, apply gentle pressure to the venepuncture site for 30–60 seconds. If the cephalic or saphenous vein was used, apply a light bandage of gauze swab or cotton wool held by cohesive bandage for 30–60 minutes.
6. Place the blood sample into the appropriate tube(s).
   - Blood should be placed in the tube containing EDTA anticoagulant last.

⟫

7. Gently invert the sample tube several times to ensure adequate distribution of any additive. Do NOT shake the tube, as this may cause haemolysis.

For bacterial culture

1–5. Follow Steps 1 to 5 above to take a 5–10 ml blood sample (see culture bottle for required volume). As a relatively large volume of blood is required, the jugular vein should be used.

6. Place a new needle on the syringe.
7. Swab the rubber stopper of the culture bottle with surgical spirit and allow to dry.
8. Add the required volume of blood to the pre-warmed culture bottle.
9. Collect three blood samples with a minimum of 1 hour between samples OR, in acutely septic patients, all three samples can be taken over 30 minutes.
10. The culture bottles should be transported to the laboratory as quickly as possible. Although not ideal, overnight postage may still give meaningful results.

Potential complications

These are very uncommon but may include:

- Minor haemorrhage
- Subcutaneous haematoma formation
- Thrombophlebitis.

Changes in serum or plasma samples

Colour	Reason for change
Pink/red	Haemolysed sample – red blood cells have been damaged due to incorrect sampling or preservation
Yellow	Icteric sample – the colour change is caused by the presence of bilirubin, which may indicate haemolytic disease, liver disease or biliary obstruction
Milky white	Lipaemic sample – due to the presence of fat in unstarved animals or evidence of liver disease

Blood smear preparation [2]

Indications/use

- Assessment of:
  - White blood cell differential count
  - Leucocyte abnormalities, e.g. toxic neutrophils, left shift, blast cells
  - Red blood cell morphology, e.g. polychromasia, anisocytosis, fragmented cells, spherocytes, Heinz bodies, parasites
  - Platelet count
  - Platelet abnormalities, e.g. macroplatelets, platelet clumps.

Equipment

- Fresh blood collected in an EDTA anticoagulant tube.
- Microhaematocrit tube.
- Microscope slides.
- A 'spreader' slide: this is narrower than the smear slide to avoid spreading the cells over the edge of the slide. 'Spreaders' can be made by breaking the corner off a normal slide, having first scored it with a blade or diamond writer.
- Hairdryer.
- Suitable stain (e.g. Diff-Quik®).
- Microscope.

Technique

Photographs reproduced from the *BSAVA Manual of Feline Practice* and courtesy of Séverine Tasker

1. Invert the EDTA tube several times to make sure the blood is well mixed. Remove a small amount of blood using a microhaemocrit tube held at a near horizontal angle.
2. Place a small drop of blood on the midline of a microscope slide, towards one end.

⏵⏵⏵

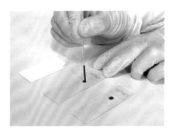

3. Hold the 'spreader' between the thumb and middle finger, placing the index finger on top of the 'spreader'.

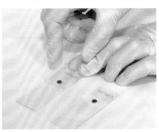

4. Place the 'spreader' in front of the blood spot, at an angle of about 30 degrees, and draw it backwards until it comes into contact with the blood, allowing the blood to spread out rapidly along the edge of the 'spreader'.

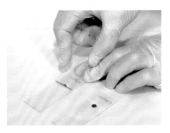

5. The moment this occurs, while keeping the 'spreader' slide at the same angle, move it rapidly yet smoothly away from you to create a blood smear.

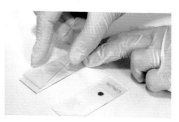

6. As the smear is made, a 'feathered edge' forms. Do not lift the 'spreader' slide until the feathered edge is complete.

7. Ideally, the smear should extend approximately two-thirds of the length of the slide.

8. Rapidly air-dry the blood smear by waving it in the air or using a hairdryer.

The smear can be sent to an external laboratory or stained in house with Romanowsky-type stains (e.g. Diff-Quik®) for routine examination.

Common faults and how to avoid them

Fault	How to avoid
Film too thick	Use a smaller drop of blood
Film too thin	Use a larger drop of blood and/or faster spreading motion
Alternating thick and thin bands	Ensure spreading motion is smooth and avoid hesitation
Streaks along length of smear	Ensure edge of spreader is not irregular or coated with dried blood Ensure no dust on slide or in blood
'Holes' in smear	Ensure slide is free of grease
Narrow, thick smear	Allow blood to spread right across spreader slide before making smear

Blood staining procedures [16]

Leishman's stain

1. Put on gloves.
2. Place slide on staining rack with smear uppermost.
3. Cover with Leishman's stain and leave for 2 minutes.
4. Add twice the stain's volume of buffered distilled water pH 6.8 and gently mix using a Pasteur pipette.
5. Leave for 10–15 minutes.
6. Wash the slide with buffered distilled water pH 6.8.
7. Allow slide to dry.

Giemsa stain

1. Put on gloves.
2. Fix the slide by dipping in methanol for 1 minute.
3. Flood the slide with diluted Giemsa stain and leave for 30 minutes.
4. Rinse the slide with distilled water.
5. Allow slide to air-dry.

Diff-Quik® stain

1. Put on gloves.
2. Dip slide into the fixative (methanol) solution (pale blue) five times for 1 second each time. Allow excess fluid to drip back into the jar.
3. Dip slide into stain (eosin) solution 1 (red) five times for 1 second each time. Allow excess fluid to drip back into the jar.
4. Dip slide into stain (methylene blue) solution 2 (purple) five times for 1 second each time. Allow excess fluid to drip back into the jar.
5. Rinse slide with distilled water.
6. Place slide vertically and leave to dry.

Blood transfusion

Collection [2, 4]

Donor selection

Changes in guidelines provided by the Royal College of Veterinary Surgeons note that the taking of blood from donors for immediate and anticipated clinical need is a recognized veterinary practice, and the UK Veterinary Medicines Directorate now permits blood banks for non-food animals following application for a specific licence. These combined changes in legislation and guidance have provided the opportunity for the development of in-house and commercial blood banking in the UK.

Dogs

- Healthy, fully vaccinated, not receiving medication (except routine endo- and ectoparasitic medications).
- Suitable temperament.
- >25 kg lean bodyweight.
- 1–8 years of age.
- Normal PCV, preferably >40%.
- Ideally DEA 1.1-negative.
- No history of a previous blood transfusion.
- Not been vaccinated within the previous 14 days.
- No history of travel outside the UK.
- Blood can be collected every 8 weeks without the need for iron supplementation.

Cats

- Healthy, fully vaccinated, not receiving medication (except routine endo- and ectoparasitic medications).
- Suitable temperament.
- >4 kg lean bodyweight.
- 1–8 years of age.
- PCV >35%.
- Blood typed (A, B or AB).
- No history of a previous blood transfusion.
- No history of travel outside the UK.

- Negative for FeLV and FIV as evaluated by a standard in-house ELISA technique.
- Negative for haemotropic *Mycoplasma* spp. evaluated by PCR.
- Blood can be collected every 8 weeks without the need for iron supplementation.

Equipment

- For aseptic preparation:
  - Regularly maintained clean, sharp electric clippers
  - Vacuum cleaner
  - Cotton wool or soft swabs
  - Container to hold used cotton wool or soft swabs
  - Tap water
  - Appropriate antiseptic
  - Appropriate sterile skin drapes.
- Blood collection containers:
  - **Dogs:** Standard commercial blood collection bag containing an anticoagulant, such as citrate phosphate dextrose (CPD), citrate phosphate dextrose adenine (CPDA) or acid citrate dextrose (ACD), attached to an extension tube and a swaged-on 16 G phlebotomy needle. These closed systems are much preferred to open systems due to the reduced potential for bacterial contamination and thus a prolonged shelf life
  - **Cats:** Three 20 ml syringes prefilled with anticoagulant (1 ml CPD, CPDA or ACD per 7.3 ml blood), a 19 or 21 G butterfly catheter or 19 G needle, 3-way tap, short extension tubing and capped needles or syringe caps.
- Topical local anaesthetic cream (e.g. EMLA cream).
- Electronic scales (for weighing blood collection bags).
- Artery forceps.
- Gauze swabs.
- Clamping device and clamps.
- Materials for a light neck bandage.

Patient preparation and positioning

- Ensure that the donor meets the criteria listed above.
- Most dogs are able to donate blood without being sedated. Cats typically require sedation.
- If required, apply topical local anaesthetic cream at least 20 minutes prior to the procedure.
- Restrain dogs securely in lateral recumbency or in a sitting position on a table.
- Restrain cats on their back with the neck extended for optimal visualization of the jugular vein; either side of the neck can be used. Alternatively, restrain the cat in lateral recumbency with the neck outstretched.

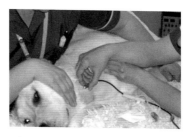

- In cats, it is advisable to preplace an intravenous catheter in a cephalic vein for the purpose of administering intravenous fluids following blood donation.
- Aseptic preparation is carried out on the skin overlying the jugular groove.

Collection procedure

Dogs

1. An assistant applies gentle pressure at the thoracic inlet to raise the jugular vein. Avoid contamination of the venepuncture site.
2. Remove the needle cap and perform venepuncture using the 16 G phlebotomy needle attached to the collection bag. If no flashback of blood is seen in the tubing, check needle placement and tubing for ➠

occlusion. The needle may need to be repositioned, but should not be fully withdrawn from the patient.

3. Position the bag lower than the donor to aid in gravitational flow and on a set of electronic scales.

4. Periodically invert the bag to ensure adequate mixing of blood and anticoagulant.

5. The maximum canine donation volume is approximately 16–18 ml/kg. The volume of blood that should be collected into a commercial blood bag is 450 ml, with an allowable 10% variance (405–495 ml). The weight of 1 ml of canine blood is approximately 1.053 g; therefore, the weight of an acceptable unit using one of these bags is approximately 426–521 g.

6. When the bag is full, clamp the tubing with a pair of artery forceps and remove the needle from the jugular vein.

7. Using a gauze swab, apply pressure over the venepuncture site for 5 minutes. A light neck bandage should be applied for several hours.

8. Strip any blood remaining in the tubing into the bag, using the fingers, inverting the bag several times to ensure adequate mixing. Allow the tubing to refill with anticoagulant blood and clamp the distal (needle) end with a hand sealer clip or heat sealer. If these are not available, a knot can be tied in the line, although this is less desirable.

9. Clamp the entire length of tubing into 10 cm segments to be used for cross-matching.

10. Label the bag with the product type, donor identification, date of collection, date of expiration, donor blood type, donor PCV and phlebotomist identification prior to use or storage.

11. Following donation, food and water can be offered. Activity should be restricted to lead walks only for the next 24 hours, and it is advised that a harness or lead passed under the chest is used instead of a neck collar and lead, to avoid pressure on the jugular venepuncture site.

Cats

1. Attach a syringe to one port of the 3-way tap and a butterfly catheter or 21 G needle to another port. A short extension tube can be attached between the 3-way tap and the butterfly catheter if required.

2. Flush the tubing with anticoagulant solution.

3. An assistant applies pressure at the thoracic inlet to raise the jugular vein. Avoid contamination of the venepuncture site.

4. Perform venepuncture using the butterfly catheter or 21 G needle. Without removing the butterfly catheter, fill each syringe in turn. The syringes can be rocked gently to ensure adequate mixing of blood and anticoagulant during collection.

5. When each syringe has been filled, close the 3-way tap, remove the syringe and place a capped needle or syringe cap on the end.

6. The maximum feline donation volume is approximately 11–13 ml/kg. When the required amount of blood has been collected, remove the butterfly needle from the vein.

7. Using a gauze swab, apply pressure over the venepuncture site for 5 minutes. A light neck bandage can be applied for several hours.

8. Label each syringe with the donor identification, blood type, time of collection and phlebotomist identification.

9. During or immediately after blood collection, 100 ml of an intravenous crystalloid should be given via the cephalic vein over 1–2 hours. The donor must be closely observed during recovery and may be offered food and water once fully awake. The donor can usually be discharged after 8–12 hours. Remove the neck bandage before sending the cat home and check the venepuncture site for bleeding.

Potential complications

- Haematoma.
- Hypovolaemic shock.

Storage

- Whole blood collected in a bag should be stored in a refrigerator maintained at 1–6°C with the bag in an upright position. Positioning the bag in this manner maximizes gas exchange with the red cell solution to help preserve the viability of the red blood cells during storage and following transfusion.
- Whole blood collected in a bag should be used within 28 days.
- Blood collected using an open system, e.g. into syringes, should be administered within 4 hours, or refrigerated and used within 24 hours.
- Whole blood can also be separated into packed red blood cells, fresh plasma, stored plasma and platelet-rich plasma concentrates. This should be done as soon as possible after collection, and plasma should be frozen within 8 hours to preserve coagulation and anticoagulation factors (fresh frozen plasma).

NOTES

Cross-matching [2]

Indications/Use

- To determine serological compatibility between a patient and donor blood.

Dogs

Cross-matching should be performed whenever:

- The recipient has received a blood transfusion >4 days previously, even if a DEA 1.1-negative donor was used
- There has been a history of transfusion reaction
- The recipient's transfusion history is unknown
- The recipient has had puppies.

Cats

Cross-matching should be performed whenever:

- The recipient requires more than one transfusion, as previously transfused blood (even though it was the same AB type) may induce antibody production against red blood cell antigens separate from the AB blood group
- The donor or recipient blood type is unknown.

Equipment

- Approximately 5 ml of blood collected in an EDTA anticoagulant tube from both the donor and recipient.
- Centrifuge.
- 5 ml plain plastic tubes.
- 0.9% saline.
- Pipette.
- Microscope slides.
- Microscope.

Patient preparation and positioning

See **Blood sampling: Venous blood sampling**

Technique

1. Collect blood from the jugular veins of the donor and recipient. Approximately 5 ml of blood from each should be placed into separate EDTA tubes. Alternatively, a sample of anticoagulated blood from the clamped sections of tubing of the blood collection bag (dogs) or collection syringes (cats) can be used.
2. Centrifuge the tubes (usually at 1000 RPM for 5–10 minutes), remove the supernatants (plasma) and transfer them to clean labelled 5 ml plain tubes (donor and recipient) for later use.
3. If a centrifuge is not available, allow the EDTA tubes to stand for ≥1 hour until the red blood cells have settled before using the supernatant.

Standard cross-match procedure

1. Wash the red blood cells three times with 0.9% saline and discard the supernatant after each wash.
2. Resuspend the washed red blood cells to create a 3–5% solution by adding 0.2 ml of red blood cells to 4.8 ml of saline (1 drop of red blood cells to 20 drops of saline).
3. For each donor prepare three tubes labelled as major, minor and recipient control.
4. To each tube add 1 drop of the appropriate 3–5% red blood cells and 2 drops of plasma according to the following:
    I.   Major cross-match = donor red blood cells and recipient plasma
    II. Minor cross-match = recipient red blood cells and donor plasma
    III. Recipient control = recipient red blood cells and recipient plasma.
5. Incubate the tubes for 15 minutes at room temperature.
6. Centrifuge the tubes at 1000 RPM for approximately 15 seconds to allow the cells to settle. Examine the

samples for haemolysis (reddening of the supernatant).

7. Gently tap the tubes to resuspend the cells. Examine and score the tubes for agglutination.

8. If macroscopic agglutination is not observed, transfer a small amount of the tube contents to a labelled glass slide and examine for microscopic agglutination. This should not be confused with rouleaux formation.

9. For the recipient control:
   i. If there is no haemolysis or agglutination in the recipient control tube, the results are valid and incompatibilities can be interpreted
   ii. If there is haemolysis or agglutination present in the recipient control tube, then the compatibility and suitability of the donor cannot be accurately assessed.

Rapid slide cross-match procedure

An alternative and more rapid, but potentially less accurate, procedure for cross-match analysis involves visualizing the presence of agglutination on a slide rather than in a tube.

1. For each donor prepare three slides labelled as major, minor and recipient control.

2. Place 1 drop of red blood cells and 2 drops of plasma on to each slide according to the following:
   i. Major cross-match = donor red blood cells and recipient plasma
   ii. Minor cross-match = recipient red blood cells and donor plasma
   iii. Recipient control = recipient red blood cells and recipient plasma.

3. Gently rock the slides to mix the plasma and red blood cells. Examine for agglutination after 1–5 minutes.

4. For the recipient control: agglutination will invalidate results.

Results of cross-matching

- Any agglutination and/or haemolysis is a 'positive' result.
- A positive **recipient control** indicates that the patient is autoagglutinating. This makes interpretation of the test difficult, although it can be repeated with additional washing of the recipient's red blood cells.
- A positive **major cross-match** indicates a significant antibody titre in the recipient against the donor red blood cells and **precludes the use of that donor for transfusions**.
- A positive **minor cross-match** indicates the presence of antibodies in the donor against the recipient red blood cells. If this reaction is strong, even small volumes of donor plasma may cause a significant transfusion reaction and precludes the use of the donor (unless red blood cells can be washed). With a weaker reaction, packed red blood cells from the donor may be transfused.

 Despite using blood products from a cross-match-compatible donor, it is still possible for a patient to experience a haemolytic or non-haemolytic transfusion reaction. Recipient monitoring during and following administration of blood products is essential.

NOTES

Blood typing [2]

Indications/Use

- **Dogs:** As DEA 1.1 is the most antigenic blood type, it is strongly advised that the DEA 1.1 status of both the donor and recipient is determined prior to transfusion, or that only DEA 1.1-negative donors are used.
- **Cats: All donor and recipient cats must be blood typed** prior to transfusion, even in an emergency situation.

Equipment

- Approximately 2 ml of blood collected into an EDTA tube.
- Blood can be submitted to a commercial laboratory for typing.
- *Alternatively*, two different commercial kits are available for in-house typing.

Dogs

- Rapid Vet-H test: This is a test card with three test 'wells' used for determining whether a dog is DEA 1.1 +ve or −ve. Two wells contain anti-DEA 1.1 antibodies, and there is also a 'control' well containing no anti-DEA 1.1 reagent. Interpretation is based on looking for the presence or absence of agglutination in the patient test well.

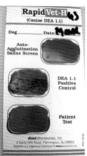

- Quick Test DEA 1.1: This migration paper strip cartridge uses monoclonal antibodies to determine whether a dog is DEA 1.1 +ve or −ve. A line adjacent to the DEA 1.1 line and the control line indicates that the dog is positive for this blood group.

Cats

- Rapid Vet-H test: This is a test card with three test 'wells': the type A well contains anti-type A reagent; the type B well contains anti-type B reagent; there is also a 'control' well containing no anti-A or

⠶⠶⠶▶

anti-B reagents. Interpretation is based on looking for an agglutination reaction in either or both test wells.

■ Quick Test A+B: This migration paper strip cartridge uses monoclonal antibodies to differentiate blood types. A line adjacent to the relevant blood group (A or B) and the control line (C) indicates the cat's blood group.

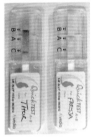

Patient preparation and positioning

See **Blood sampling: Venous blood sampling**

Technique

Use a commercial blood typing test kit and follow manufacturer's instructions.

■ Care should be taken when blood typing severely anaemic dogs and cats. The *prozone effect* (due to the low number of red blood cells, the quantity of antigen is reduced compared with the amount of antibody in the reagent) may prevent proper agglutination of blood with the reagent. It may be helpful to centrifuge the whole blood sample and remove one drop of the plasma, to increase the relative concentration of red blood cells. The red blood cells and plasma are then remixed prior to performing the blood typing test.

■ Despite using blood products from a blood-typed donor, it is still possible for a patient to experience a haemolytic or non-haemolytic transfusion reaction. Recipient monitoring during and following administration of blood products is essential.

Administering the blood [2]

Indications/Use

- Anaemia.
- Coagulopathies, although consideration should be given to the use of fresh frozen plasma or cryoprecipitate. Note, however, that stored blood will be severely depleted in several clotting factors.
- Preparation for anticipated blood loss during surgery.

Contraindications

- Administration of non-typed or non-cross-matched blood to a dog that has previously received a blood transfusion.
- Administration of non-typed blood to a cat.

Equipment

- For intravenous catheter placement:
  - Over-the-needle intravenous catheter, comprising a needle (or stylet) with a catheter fitted over the needle
  - No. 11 scalpel
  - T-connector or extension set containing heparinized saline (1 IU of heparin per ml of 0.9% saline), or injection cap
  - Adhesive tape
  - Soft padded bandage and outer protective bandage
  - Appropriate skin antiseptic.
- Whole blood:
  - **Dogs:** As a general rule:
    - DEA 1.1-negative dogs should only receive DEA 1.1-negative blood
    - DEA 1.1-positive dogs may receive either DEA 1.1-negative or -positive blood
  - **Cats:**
    - Type A cats must only receive type A blood
    - Type B cats must only receive type B blood

▭▶

- The rarer type AB cats do not possess either alloantibody; they should ideally receive type AB blood, but when this is not available type A blood is the next best choice, followed by type B blood.

INSPECTION OF BLOOD

Visual inspection of the blood is necessary prior to administration. Discoloration (brown, purple), the presence of clots or haemolysis may indicate bacterial contamination and the blood should not be used.

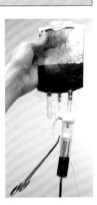

- **Dogs:** Blood infusion set incorporating an in-line filter (170–260 μm) and suitable for connecting to a canine blood collection bag.
- **Cats:** A plain 150 ml blood collection bag and blood giving set with in-line filter (170–260 μm). All the blood collected into the syringes is injected slowly into the plain blood collection bag through the injection port.

Alternatively, blood collected into syringes can be administered via an extension set using a syringe driver. Again a filter should be used, such as a paediatric filter with reduced dead space or micro-aggregate filters of 18–40 μm.

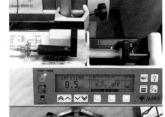

- The intravenous catheter should be suitable for the size of the patient. A large-diameter catheter should be placed to avoid red cell haemolysis during blood administration.

Patient preparation and positioning

- The patient should ideally be conscious, although sedation can be used if required. It is sometimes necessary to give blood to an anaesthetized patient intraoperatively.

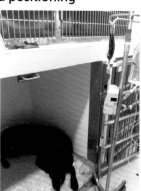

- The patient should be placed on comfortable bedding.
- Patients should not receive food or medication during a transfusion, and the only fluid that may be administered through the same catheter is 0.9% saline.
- The intravenous catheter should be placed in a peripheral vein. Alternatively, blood can be given via an intraosseous cannula if venous access cannot be obtained.

Technique

- Blood is usually administered intravenously via an intravenous catheter, but it may also be given via the intraosseous route if venous access cannot be obtained (e.g. kittens, puppies). It should not be given intraperitoneally.
- Blood does not need to be warmed prior to use, unless being given to neonates or other very small animals. Warming may lead to haemolysis of red cells, as well as providing favourable conditions for proliferation of any microbial contaminant.

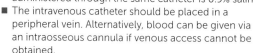

- Care should be taken if blood is administered to patients with increased risk of volume overload (e.g. cardiovascular disease, impaired renal function).
- Blood should not be given through a catheter that contains, or has contained without flushing, calcium-containing fluids.

Volume

The amount of blood to be administered can be calculated as follows:

- As a 'rule of thumb':
  - 2 ml blood/kg bodyweight raises the PCV by 1%
- Suggested formulae for calculating the amount of whole blood required for transfusion are:
  - **Dog:**
    Volume of donor blood required = recipient's bodyweight (kg) x 85 x

    $$\frac{\text{desired PCV} - \text{recipient's PCV}}{\text{PCV of donated blood}}$$

  - **Cat:**
    Volume of donor blood required = recipient's bodyweight (kg) x 60 x

    $$\frac{\text{desired PCV} - \text{recipient's PCV}}{\text{PCV of donated blood}}$$

Total volume given should not exceed 22 ml/kg unless there are severe ongoing losses.

Rate

The rate of whole blood administration depends on the cardiovascular status of the recipient:

- In general, the rate should be only 0.25–1.0 ml/kg/h for the first 20–30 minutes
- If the transfusion is well tolerated, the rate may then be increased to around 5–10 ml/kg/h, aiming to deliver the remaining product within 4 hours. *Blood should not be administered over a period longer than*

*4 hours owing to the increased risk of bacterial
proliferation within the product*
- In an animal with an increased risk of volume overload
  (cardiovascular disease, impaired renal function), the
  rate of administration should not exceed 3–4 ml/kg/h.

 Fluid pumps should NOT be used for
RBC transfusions unless they have been
validated appropriately for such use by the
manufacturer, because they could induce
red cell haemolysis.

Monitoring

Continuous monitoring during the transfusion is required
for signs of a reaction.

- The following parameters should be recorded prior to
  the transfusion ('baseline'), every 5 minutes during the
  first 30 minutes of the transfusion, and then every 15
  minutes for the remainder of the transfusion:
    - Demeanour
    - Rectal temperature
    - Pulse rate and quality
    - Respiratory rate and character
    - Mucous membrane colour and capillary refill
      time
    - Plasma and urine colour.
- PCV and TP should also be monitored prior to, upon
  completion of, and at 12 and 24 hours after
  transfusion.

NOTES

Adverse reactions [2]

Acute haemolytic reaction with intravascular haemolysis

- Seen in type B cats receiving type A blood, as well as in DEA 1.1-negative dogs sensitized to DEA 1.1 upon repeated exposure.
- Clinical signs may include fever, tachycardia, dyspnoea, muscle tremors, vomiting, weakness, collapse, haemoglobinaemia and haemoglobinuria.
- May lead to shock, disseminated intravascular coagulation, renal damage and, potentially, death.
- **Treatment involves immediate discontinuation of the transfusion** and treatment of the clinical signs of shock.

Non-haemolytic immunological reactions

- Acute type I hypersensitivity reactions (allergic or anaphylactic), most often mediated by IgE and mast cells.
- Clinical signs include urticaria, pruritus, erythema, oedema, vomiting and dyspnoea secondary to pulmonary oedema.
- **Treatment involves immediate discontinuation of the transfusion** and evaluation of the patient for evidence of haemolysis and shock. Steroids (dexamethasone 0.5–1.0 mg/kg i.v.) and antihistamines (chlorphenamine 4–8 mg q8h for dogs; 2–4 mg q8–12h for cats) may be required.

NOTES

NOTES

Body condition scoring scheme — cats [21]

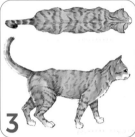

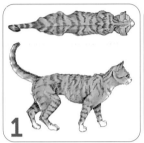

Under ideal

1. Ribs visible on shorthaired cats. No palpable fat. Severe abdominal tuck. Lumbar vertebrae and wings of ilia easily palpated.
2. Ribs easily visible on shorthaired cats. Lumbar vertebrae obvious. Pronounced abdominal tuck. No palpable fat.
3. Ribs easily palpable with minimal fat covering. Lumbar vertebrae obvious. Obvious waist behind ribs. Minimal abdominal fat.

Ideal

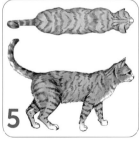

4. Ribs palpable with minimal fat covering. Noticeable waist behind ribs. Slight abdominal tuck. Abdominal fat pad absent.
5. Well-proportioned. Observe waist behind ribs. Ribs palpable with slight fat covering. Abdominal fat pad minimal.

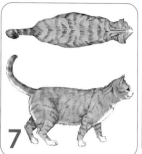
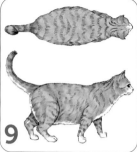

Over ideal

6. Ribs palpable with slight excess fat covering. Waist and abdominal fat pad distinguishable but not obvious. Abdominal tuck absent.

7. Ribs not easily palpated with moderate fat covering. Waist poorly discernible. Obvious rounding of abdomen. Moderate abdominal fat pad.

8. Ribs not palpable with excess fat covering. Waist absent. Obvious rounding of abdomen with prominent abdominal fat pad. Fat deposits present over lumbar area.

9. Ribs not palpable under heavy fat cover. Heavy fat deposits over lumbar area, face and limbs. Distention of abdomen with no waist. Extensive abdominal fat deposits.

Courtesy of WSAVA Global
Nutrition Committee

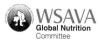

Body condition scoring scheme – dogs [21]

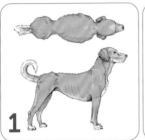

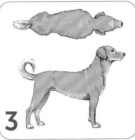

Under ideal

1. Ribs, lumbar vertebrae, pelvic bones and all bony prominences evident from a distance. No discernible body fat. Obvious loss of muscle mass.
2. Ribs, lumbar vertebrae and pelvic bones easily visible. No palpable fat. Some evidence of other bony prominences. Minimal loss of muscle mass.
3. Ribs easily palpated and maybe visible with no palpable fat. Tops of lumbar vertebrae visible. Pelvic bones becoming prominent. Obvious waist and abdominal tuck.

Ideal

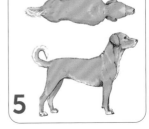

4. Ribs easily palpable, with minimal fat covering. Waist easily noted, viewed from above. Abdominal tuck evident.
5. Ribs palpable without excess fat covering. Waist observed behind ribs when viewed from above. Abdomen tucked up when viewed from side.

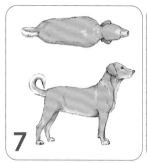

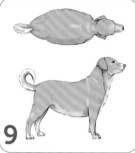

7

9

Over ideal

6. Ribs palpable with slight excess fat covering. Waist is discernible viewed from above but is not prominent. Abdominal tuck apparent.

7. Ribs palpable with difficulty; heavy fat cover. Noticeable fat deposits over lumbar area and base of tail. Waist absent or barely visible. Abdominal tuck may be present.

8. Ribs not palpable under very heavy fat cover, or palpable only with significant pressure. Heavy fat deposits over lumbar area and base of tail. Waist absent. No abdominal tuck. Obvious abdominal distention may be present.

9. Massive fat deposits over thorax, spine and base of tail. Waist and abdominal tuck absent. Fat deposits on neck and limbs. Obvious abdominal distention.

Courtesy of WSAVA Global Nutrition Committee

WSAVA
Global Nutrition
Committee

Body condition scoring scheme – rabbits

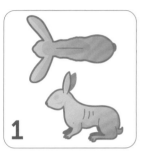

Very thin

More than 20% below ideal body weight

- Hip bones, ribs and spine are very sharp to the touch
- Loss of muscle and no fat cover
- The rump area curves in

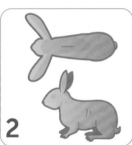

Thin

Between 10–20% below ideal body weight

- Hip bones, ribs and spine are easily felt
- Loss of muscle and very little fat cover
- Rump area is flat

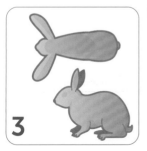

Ideal

- Hip bones, ribs and spine are easily felt but are rounded, not sharp – ribs feel like a pocket full of pens!
- No abdominal bulge
- Rump area is flat

Overweight

10–15% above ideal body weight

- Pressure is needed to feel the ribs, spine and hip bones
- Some fat layers
- The rump is rounded

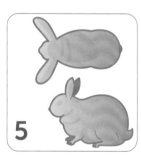

Obese

More than 15% above ideal body weight

- Very hard to feel the spine and hip bones – ribs cannot be felt!
- Tummy sags with obvious fat padding
- Rump bulges out

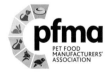

Illustrations are taken from the Pet Food Manufacturers' Association Rabbit-Size-O-Meter with their permission. For more information, please visit **www.pfma.org.uk**

Calculating blood loss [16]

Two methods of estimating blood loss are provided below. When using either technique, remember to subtract the volume of any lavage fluids that have been used and that have also been soaked up by the swabs.

1. Collect all used swabs.
2. Count them.
3. Weigh them.
4. Weigh the same number of dry new swabs (if only a couple of swabs have been used weigh 10 swabs and then divide the weight by 10 and multiply by the number used).
5. Subtract the weight of the dry new swabs from the weight of the used, bloody swabs.
6. Calculate the weight of blood contained in the swabs, assuming 1 g equates to 1 ml of fluid/blood.
7. Measure any blood in suction containers and estimate the blood on the floor, drapes and surgeon.
8. Establish the volume of any saline or other fluids used by the surgeon.
9. Add together the volume of blood loss calculated from the swabs, suction, etc., and subtract the volume of any other fluids used by the surgeon to establish the total volume of blood lost.
10. Estimate the patient's blood volume (88 ml x bodyweight (kg) in the dog, 66 ml x bodyweight (kg) in the cat).
11. Divide the estimated blood volume by 100 and multiply by the estimated blood loss (ml).
12. This equates to % blood loss compared to the total blood volume of the patient.

NOTES

EXAMPLE

A 25 kg dog is anaesthetized for ovariohysterectomy. During ligation of the second ovary the ligature around the ovarian pedicle slips and the abdomen starts to fill with blood. The veterinary surgeon gains control of the bleeding after a few minutes but uses a large number of swabs to soak up the haemorrhage. You are concerned about blood loss and wish to calculate the % blood loss in this patient.

1. Ask the surgeon to put the used swabs from the surgical trolley into a container.
2. Count the number of used swabs and find it is 15 small swabs.
3. Weigh a dry swab (6 g) and calculate the weight of the used swabs when dry (6 g x 15 = 90 g).
4. Weigh the used swabs and read off the total weight from the scale. In this case it is 375 g.
5. Calculate the weight of blood in the used swabs (375–90 = 285 g).
6. 1 g of blood is roughly the weight of 1 ml of blood so the total amount of blood lost is 285 ml.
7. The blood volume of a 25 kg dog is 25 x 88 ml = 2,200 ml or 2.2 l.
8. The percentage blood loss in this patient is 285/2,200 x 100 = 12.95%.
9. This percentage blood loss would indicate that fluid therapy with a polyionic solution is indicated to replace blood volume.

Alternatively, a good estimate of the patient's blood loss can be calculated using the following technique:

1. Find out the volume of water needed to saturate 10 swabs.
2. Divide this by 10 for the volume of water needed to saturate one swab.

3. This is roughly equivalent to the volume of blood that will be contained in one swab.
4. Multiply the volume of blood contained in one saturated swab by the number of swabs used in the surgery to estimate the volume of blood lost.

EXAMPLE

If 10 swabs will absorb 50 ml of water, one swab will absorb 5 ml. During an operation, 14 swabs become saturated in blood. An estimate of the volume of blood soaked into these swabs is 70 ml (14 x 5).

See also **Blood transfusion**

Catheterization *see* **Intravenous catheter management, Urinary catheters**

NOTES

Cleaning the operating theatre[16]

At the beginning of each day

- All the surfaces, furniture and equipment in the theatre suite should be damp-dusted, using a dilute solution of disinfectant (a dry duster would simply move dust around the room). Damp-dusting is performed to remove any traces of dust particles that may have settled overnight on the surfaces and equipment within the theatre. Starting at the top and working downwards helps ensure all dust is removed.

Between cases

- The operating table, stands, instrument trolleys, kick buckets, monitoring equipment and leads should be wiped clean using an appropriate disinfectant.
- The floors should be mopped clean. The operating table should be moved to allow cleaning if the floor has become contaminated with any fluid during a procedure.
- The scrub sink area, including the adjacent wall, should be cleaned.
- All waste material should be removed and disposed of appropriately.

At the end of the day

- The floors in all rooms of the theatre suite should be vacuumed or swept to remove debris and loose hair. The vacuum and hose should be emptied and thoroughly cleaned.
- The floors should then be either wet-vacuumed or washed using disinfectant.
- All waste material should be removed and disposed of.
- Surfaces, equipment, operating tables, lights and scrub sinks should all be thoroughly washed down with disinfectant.

Once a week

- There should be a more thorough deep cleaning session of the operating theatres.
- All equipment should be removed from the room and the floors and walls should then be scrubbed.
- A disinfectant with detergent properties that will remove organic matter and that is active against a wide range of bacteria, including *Pseudomonas* spp., should be used.
- After removing any excess solution, the disinfectant should be allowed to dry on the surface rather than being rinsed off, for longer residual activity.
- All equipment should be meticulously wiped over with disinfectant.

Once a month

- All air vents should be vacuumed and cleaned thoroughly to remove any dust build-up.

NOTES

Clinical audits [16, 20]

A clinical audit is a process used to assess, evaluate and reflect on the effectiveness of a procedure in a systematic way in order to improve patient care and outcomes. Audits should be part of a continuous quality improvement process that focuses on specific problems or aspects of clinical practice. A specific area of clinical practice is selected, data are collected and compared with 'best practice' and evidence-based research in order to make a decision on whether protocols are reaching the correct standard or if modifications are required. Examples of clinical audits used in practice include those for:

- Antimicrobial resistance (*see* **PROTECT ME**)
- Blood pressure monitoring (*see* **Blood pressure measurement**)
- Client compliance in postoperative care
- Incidence of postoperative hypothermia
- Indwelling devices (*see* **Urinary catheters**)
- Infection control and hygiene (*see* **Infection control**)
- Pain scoring and analgesia (*see* **Pain assessment**)
- Postoperative wound care (*see* **Wound drain management**)
- Significant events
- Prescription medication dispensing errors.

Useful websites for further reading

RCVS Knowledge:
  www.rcvsknowledge.org/quality-improvement
vetAUDIT:
  https://vetaudit.rcvsk.org
BSAVA Library:
- BSAVA Guide to the Use of Veterinary Medicines: www.bsavalibrary.com/medicinesguide
- Congress Proceedings 2019: Clinical audit: how to set up https://www.bsavalibrary.com/content/congress

Dental recording chart — cat[8]

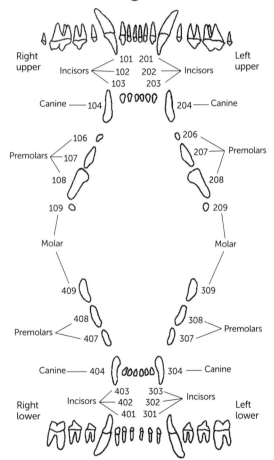

Right upper

Incisors — 101 201 — Incisors

102 202

103 203

Canine — 104 204 — Canine

Left upper

Premolars — 106 206 — Premolars

107 207

108 208

109 209

Molar — — Molar

409 309

408 308

Premolars — 407 307 — Premolars

Canine — 404 304 — Canine

Right lower

Incisors — 403 303 — Incisors

402 302

401 301

Left lower

(Courtesy of Alexander M. Reiter, Dentistry and Oral Surgery Service, School of Veterinary Medicine, University of Pennsylvania)

Dental recording chart – dog [8]

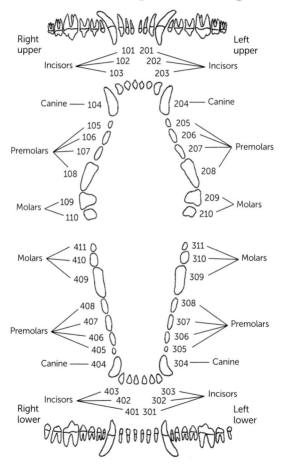

Right upper

Left upper

Incisors — 101 201 — Incisors
102 202
103 203

Canine — 104 204 — Canine

Premolars — 105 205 — Premolars
106 206
107 207
108 208

Molars — 109 209 — Molars
110 210

Molars — 411 311 — Molars
410 310
409 309

Premolars — 408 308 — Premolars
407 307
406 306
405 305

Canine — 404 304 — Canine

Incisors — 403 303 — Incisors
402 302
401 301

Right lower

Left lower

(Courtesy of Alexander M. Reiter, Dentistry and Oral Surgery Service, School of Veterinary Medicine, University of Pennsylvania)

NOTES

Ear cytology[7]

Samples are usually taken from the ears to identify parasites or cells and microorganisms. Samples should be collected after an initial otoscopic examination, but before cleaning. A cotton bud is inserted down to the junction between the vertical and horizontal ear canals and rotated to collect debris, which is transferred on to a slide for cytology. The debris can be mixed with liquid paraffin, a coverslip applied and the slide examined. Under low power (X4 objective), *Otodectes*, *Demodex*, their eggs and plant debris are easily visible, but a higher magnification (the X40 or X100 lens) is required to see yeasts or bacteria clearly. Sterile swabs used to collect material can be submitted in transport medium for bacterial culture.

NOTES

Ear cytology findings and their significance

Finding	Description	Significance
Keratinocytes	Large, flat and angular. Stain pale blue to pale purple. May have melanin or keratohyaline granules. Occasionally nucleated	Shed keratinocytes; normal
	Large trapezoid to cigar shapes. Stain deep purple–blue	Shed keratinocytes; normal
	Large flat, angular to round, nucleated cells. Stain deep purple–blue	Acanthocytes; pemphigus foliaceus but also seen in severe bacterial infections
	Polymorphic nucleus and pale cytoplasm	Associated with infection, inflammation and ulceration (see also red blood cells)
Neutrophils	Large nucleus, open and disrupted chromatin pattern (karyorrhexis). Often see nuclear streaming	Degenerate (or toxic) neutrophils; a good indication of infection
	Dark, shrunken nucleus (pyknosis). Nuclear streaming uncommon	Non-degenerate neutrophils; an indication of sterile inflammation
	Intracytoplasmic bacteria	Definite indicator of infection rather than bacterial contamination

Finding	Description	Significance
Malassezia	Large ovoid to budding yeasts	Low numbers (<5 per high power field) probably normal in most dogs; larger numbers suggest *Malassezia* otitis
Bacteria	Small cocci, often in groups. Blue to purple stain	Staphylococci; low numbers probably normal in most dogs, larger numbers suggest bacterial overgrowth and otitis. More serious infections associated with neutrophils
	Small, short rods; blue to purple stain. Usually with degenerate neutrophils	Gram-negative rods, usually *Pseudomonas*; these are not seen in healthy ears and are therefore clinically significant
Red blood cells	Small, round anucleate cells	Haemorrhage, associated with trauma and ulceration

Electrocardiography [2, 4]

Obtaining an electrocardiogram

1. Place patient on a dry insulated surface.
2. Use standard positioning if this is not too distressing for the patient.
3. Attach one electrode on each limb in the standard configuration (Einthoven's limb lead system): on the forelimbs just above or below the olecranon; and on the hindlimbs just above or below the stifle. Electrodes can be stainless steel crocodile clips or adhesive patches (adhesive patch electrodes are best for long-term monitoring). Electrode jelly is used with clips to improve skin contact. Surgical spirit may be used but needs regular application as it evaporates. Do not allow the electrodes to contact each other, and keep the patient as still as possible during the procedure.
4. Record 5–10 complexes of leads I, II, III, aVr, aVl and aVf at paper speed 25 mm/second.
5. Record a rhythm strip of lead II at paper speed 50 mm/second.

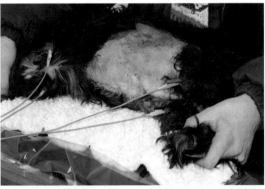

Standard positioning for a diagnostic ECG. The dog is restrained in right lateral recumbency with the limbs extended.

6. Run a longer rhythm strip at a slower speed if possible when checking for dysrhythmia.
7. Record patient details, date, position and any drugs administered for reference.
8. Make a note of the paper speed, calibration (cm:mV) and whether filters were used.

Standard leads for electrocardiography

Lead	Attachment site	Colour
RA ('right arm')	Right elbow	Red
LA ('left arm')	Left elbow	Yellow
F or LL ('left leg')	Left stifle	Green
N or RL ('right leg', earth lead)	Right stifle	Black

Lead II at 1 cm/mV and 50 mm/s

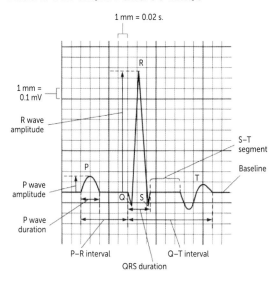

NOTES

Faecal examination[13]

Indications	Method
Gross examination	
Preliminary assessment	Assess: • Consistency and colour • Presence of mucus or fat • Presence of specific material (worms, foreign material, undigested food)
Direct smear	
Parasitic burden Undigested starch or muscle fibres	1. Place one drop of saline and one drop of faeces on slide. 2. Mix thoroughly; remove any large pieces of faecal material. 3. Smear and heat-fix, or cover with a coverslip. 4. Stain by placing a drop of stain at corner of coverslip and allow to spread. 5. Use 2% Lugol's iodine for starch (blue–black). 6. Use eosin, new methylene blue, Wright's for undigested muscle fibres. 7. Look for worm eggs under low power and protozoa under medium power.
Faecal flotation	
Worm eggs Protozoa	Mix faeces with saturated sugar or zinc sulphate ($ZnSO_4$) solution[a]. (Note: Zinc sulphate flotation must be used for *Giardia* as other suspensions will cause destruction of this organism.) 8. Ova and cysts will rise to surface, but centrifugation will improve sensitivity. 9. Examine supernatant within 15 minutes if looking for *Giardia*.
Faecal fat	
Undigested fat	1. Mix one drop of fresh faeces with one drop of Sudan III on a glass slide. 2. Examine microscopically. 3. Undigested fat will be seen as orange droplets.

[a] $ZnSO_4$ solution is made by mixing 331 grams of $ZnSO_4$ in 1 litre of water.

Feeding tube selection [13]

Indications	Contraindications	
Naso-oesophageal tube		
Anorexia. Oral food intake reduced for more than 3 days. Loss of >5% bodyweight. Where a general anaesthetic is contraindicated. When long-term enteral feeding is required (7–10 days)	Non-functional gastrointestinal tract, oesophageal disease, persistent vomiting, unconsciousness	
Orogastric (stomach) tube		
Usually repeated tube placement, not indwelling. When rapid feeding is required. For neonates during first few days of life. Anorexia in exotic species. Particularly useful in chelonians suffering from post-hibernation anorexia	Oral trauma, pharyngeal trauma	
Pharyngostomy tube		
Facial, mandibular or maxillary disease, trauma or surgery. Long-term support required	Pharyngeal trauma, non-functional gastrointestinal tract, persistent vomiting, unconsciousness	

Complications	Advantages	Disadvantages
Occlusion of the tube. Regurgitation of the tube (particularly in cats). Patient interference. Ingestion of part of the tube. Diarrhoea (due to bacterial overgrowth or increased water intake, or feeding too quickly)	Easy to place. Can be used for up to a week. Animal still able to eat and drink with tube in place. Inexpensive	Small-gauge tube so only certain liquid feeds can be used
Aspiration pneumonia if tube is misplaced. Mouth must be kept open throughout feeding to prevent patient from chewing the tube	Useful in neonates and exotics. Relatively easy procedure. Can be placed whilst animal is conscious. Requires little or no maintenance	Not well tolerated by adults. Short-term use only – can be used for 2–3 days. Requires cooperative patient as the tube is passed
Interference with epiglottal function. Oedema. Infection at site of skin puncture. Haemorrhage. Occlusion of the tube. Aspiration of food. Patient interference	Useful for short- to mid-term use. Easy to administer any liquidized food into the oesophagus	Requires general anaesthesia so unsuitable for weak/unstable animals. Can be easily dislodged. Stoma site can become infected. Limited to liquid diets. Most useful for short-term feeding (<14 days). May induce gagging. Can be associated with partial airway obstruction

Indications	Contraindications	
Gastrostomy tube; percutaneous endoscopically placed gastrostomy (PEG) tube		
Upper gastrointestinal tract must be bypassed. Anorexic patients. Placed either surgically, by endoscopy, or percutaneously	Malabsorption in digestive tract, non-functional gastrointestinal tract, persistent vomiting	
Jejunostomy tube		
Upper gastrointestinal tract must be bypassed. Long-term support required	Non-functional lower gastrointestinal tract, malabsorption	

NOTES

Complications	Advantages	Disadvantages
Hyperglycaemia. Occlusion of the tube. Infection at site of skin puncture. Patient interference. Peritonitis	Large-diameter tube. Easy to feed. Any liquidized food may be fed. Can be left *in situ* for months at a time; special low-profile tubes available for prolonged feeding. Patient tolerance excellent	Requires general anaesthesia. Specialized equipment required (endoscope). Should remain in place for minimum of 5–7 days to ensure adequate adhesions form between stomach and abdominal wall
Infection. Digestive tract complications	Can be used long term.	Requires general anaesthesia. Predigested and very simple nutritional units must be delivered to avoid severe digestive tract complications. Prolonged hospitalization usually required. Expensive. High maintenance

NOTES

Feeding tubes — nursing considerations[4]

Managing patients with feeding tubes requires special attention. Oesophagostomy, gastrostomy and jejunostomy tubes are secured in place with sutures and the tubes are then bandaged. The dressings and bandages should be inspected daily for any sign of infection and the site cleaned. After each use, all feeding tubes should be flushed with water to prevent clogging. Prevention of premature removal of tubes can be accomplished by using Elizabethan collars and by bandaging tubes securely. Care should be taken to avoid wrapping too tightly as this could lead to patient discomfort and even compromise proper ventilation.

As enteral diets are mostly composed of water (most canned foods are already >75% water) the amount of fluids administered parenterally should be adjusted accordingly to avoid volume overload.

The majority of complications from feeding tubes involve tube occlusion or localized irritation at the tube exit site. More serious complications include infection at the exit site or, rarely, complete tube dislodgment and peritonitis (gastrostomy or jejunostomy tube).

Complications can be avoided by using the appropriate tube, effectively securing the tube, proper diet selection and preparation, and careful monitoring.

Formulating an enteral feeding plan

1. **Calculate patient's resting energy requirement (RER)**
   RER (kcal to feed per day) = 70 × (bodyweight)$^{0.75}$ or
   30 × (bodyweight) + 70 if bodyweight 2–30 kg
   For the first day, feed only 50% of the RER.

2. Select diet, based on type of tube to be used

Tube type	Appropriate diets
Naso-oesophageal	Use liquid diets, e.g. Royal Canin Recovery Liquid (Dog & Cat)
Oesophagostomy	For tubes >14 Fr, use liquid diets For tubes up to 14 Fr, can use convalescence support instant diets
Gastrostomy	Can use more concentrated diets, e.g. convalescence support instant diets; Hill's a/d; blended maintenance diets
Jejunostomy	Liquid diets only

3a. Using complete liquid diets

For example, Royal Canin Recovery Liquid (Dog & Cat): contains 1 kcal/ml.

From known RER for patient, calculate ml required daily.

May be better tolerated as constant rate infusion in sick patients at 0.5–0.6 ml/kg/h.

3b. Using convalescence support instant diets

For example, Convalescence Canine/Feline Instant: contains 473 kcal/100 g (4.73 kcal/g). *Note: this is very high in protein (8.9 g/100 kcal) and sodium (80 mg/100 kcal) and may therefore be unsuitable for patients with hepatic encephalopathy or congestive heart failure.*

From known RER for patient, calculate grams required daily.

To reconstitute: Use one part diet (grams) to three parts water (mililitres) to allow easy passage down an oesophagostomy tube (14 Fr with the exit site made bigger) – this will have 1.2 kcal/ml.

Divide into 3–6 feedings per day.

Fine needle aspiration of a mass[2,13]

1. Lay out at least five slides on a clean surface and draw back an empty 10 ml syringe.
2. Clip the area to be aspirated and clean with spirit.
3. Immobilize the mass if possible (aspirates of body organs should be performed with ultrasound guidance).

Needle-only technique

1. Insert the needle into the mass and move it rapidly in and out (to ensure cells are broken away from the tissue).
2. Remove the needle and attach to a syringe containing 10 ml of air.

Fine needle aspiration with suction

1. With the needle attached to the syringe, insert the needle into the mass.
2. Draw back on the syringe to the 5 ml mark (this should be quite difficult because of negative pressure created).
3. Whilst maintaining suction, move the needle around within the mass.
4. Release suction before removing the needle from the mass.
5. Remove needle from end of syringe, draw 10 ml air into the syringe and reattach to the needle.

Making the smear

1. With the bevel of the needle facing down, squirt out the contents of the needle on to one end of a clean slide.
2. Make a smear or a squash preparation.

Squash preparation

With experience, this technique produces excellent smears. However, in inexperienced hands cells may be damaged/ruptured, resulting in an unreadable smear.

1. Expel the aspirate on to the centre of a microscope slide.

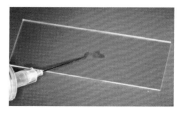

2. Place a second spreader slide horizontally and at right angles to spread the sample, taking care not to exert downward pressure that could rupture the cells.
3. Using only the surface tension between the two slides, draw the spreader slide quickly and smoothly across the bottom slide.

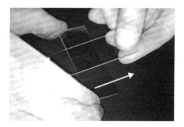

4. Rapidly dry the smear by waving it in the air or under a hairdryer. **Note that it is the smear produced on the *underside of the spreader slide* that will be examined.**

Fluid therapy[13, 16]

Clinical signs of dehydration

Dehydration level	Clinical signs
<5%	• Not detectable
5–6%	• Subtle loss of skin elasticity
6–8%	• Marked loss of skin elasticity • Slightly prolonged capillary refill time • Slightly sunken eyes • Dry mucous membranes
10–12%	• Tented skin stands in place • Capillary refill time >2 seconds • Sunken eyes • Dry mucous membranes
12–15%	• Early shock • Moribund • Death imminent

Calculating fluid loss using PCV

If a 4.5 kg dehydrated cat has a PCV of 43%, how much fluid can it be estimated has been lost?

- Normal cat PCV = 35%
- Current PCV = 43%
- Increase = 8%
- For every 1% increase in PCV, animal requires 10 ml fluid/kg
- 8% increase in PCV = 8 x 10 ml x 4.5 kg = 360 ml

Answer: 360 ml of fluid

Calculating fluid loss using bodyweight

Prior to illness, a Border Terrier weighed 12 kg. Following an episode of vomiting and diarrhoea, the same animal was found to weigh 11.2 kg. How much fluid can it be estimated to have lost?

- Difference in bodyweight = 12 − 11.2 = 0.8 kg (800 g)
- 1 kg = 1 litre, therefore 800 g = 800 ml

Answer: 800 ml

Estimating fluid loss due to known losses

Often, ongoing losses will need to be estimated. One episode of vomiting or diarrhoea can be estimated as 4 ml/kg fluid loss. A 12 kg dog has vomited twice and had one episode of diarrhoea. Estimate the fluid loss.

- Vomit = 2 x 4 ml/kg x 12 kg = 96 ml
- Diarrhoea = 1 x 4 ml/kg x 12 kg = 48 ml
- Total = 144 ml

Calculating fluid rates

A 20 kg Border Collie with vomiting and diarrhoea is estimated to be 8% dehydrated. The giving set delivers 20 drops/ml. Calculate the rate of drops per minute.

The aim is to replace any fluid deficits over 24 hours, so the total daily requirement is:

Replacement of losses + Maintenance requirements + Ongoing losses

1. Fluid deficit (ml) = bodyweight (kg) x % dehydration x 10
   20 x 8 x 10 = 1600 ml
2. Maintenance requirement = 50 ml/kg/day
   50 x 20 = 1000 ml/day
3. Estimate ongoing losses:
   - Diarrhoea: 5 episodes at 4 ml/kg = 400 ml/day
   - Vomiting: 5 episodes at 4 ml/kg = 400 ml/day
   - Total ongoing losses = 800 ml/day
4. Daily requirement = deficit + maintenance + ongoing losses
   1600 + 1000 + 800 = 3400 ml/day
5. Hourly fluid requirement = 3400 ÷ 24 = 142 ml/h
6. Drop rate = 142 x 20 = 2840 drops/h
   2840 ÷ 60 = 47 drops/minute

Bolus doses of fluids for hypovolaemic patients

Degree of hypovolaemia	Bolus dose: dogs	Bolus dose: cats
Mild	5–10 ml/kg	3–5 ml/kg
Moderate	10–20 ml/kg	5–10 ml/kg
Severe	20–40 ml/kg (may need repeating)	10–15 ml/kg (may need repeating)

Crystalloid solutions

Crystalloid solution	Na^+ (mmol/l)	K^+ (mmol/l)	Cl^- (mmol/l)	Ca^{2+} mmol/l	Tonicity relative to extracellular fluid
Replacement					
Hartmann's solution	131	5	111	2	Isotonic
Lactated Ringer's solution	130	4	109	1.5	Isotonic
0.9% NaCl ('normal' saline)	154	0	154	0	Isotonic
Maintenance					
0.45% NaCl + 2.5% dextrose (glucose)	77	0	77	0	Hypotonic
Normosol-M + 5% dextrose (glucose)	40	13	40	0	Mildly hypotonic
Others					
0.45% NaCl (half strength saline)	77	0	77	0	Hypotonic
0.9% NACl + 5% glucose	154	0	154	0	Hypertonic
7.2% NaCl (hypertonic saline)	1232	0	1232	0	Hypertonic

Colloid solutions

Colloid type	Example product names	Duration of action	Rate of fluid administration
Gelatins	Gelofusine	Up to 6 hours	Maximum dose: 20 ml/kg/24 hours
Starch (hetastarch, pentastarch)	elo-HAES, HAES-steril, Hemohes, Voluven, Volulyte	24–36 hours	Maximum dose: 20 ml/kg/24 hours

NOTES

Folding gowns and drapes[16]

Folding a gown

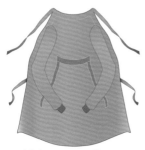

(1) Lay gown flat out.

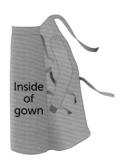

(2) Fold side to middle.

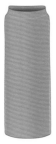

(3) Fold over other side to edge.

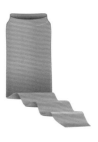

(4) Concertina lengthways.

(5) Pick up by inside of collar after autoclaving.

Folding surgical drapes

(1, 2) Concertina cloth widthways.   (2)

(3) Concertina lengthways.

(4) Pack cloths in autoclave drum or autoclave bags sealed with indicating tape.

Folding a plain drape

1. The drape is folded in half widthways

2–4. It is then folded in half lengthways three times, so that there are two corners at the top

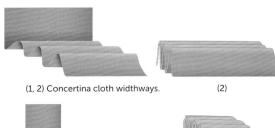

Gowning and gloving[16]

Putting on a surgical gown

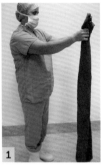

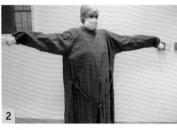

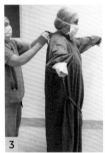

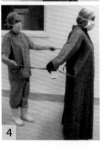

1. The sterile gown (folded inside out) is taken from its sterile pack, held at the shoulders and allowed to fall open.
2. One hand is slipped into each sleeve. No attempt should be made to try to pull the sleeves over the shoulder or to readjust the gown, as this will lead to contamination of the hands or outside of the gown.
3. An unscrubbed assistant should pull the back of the gown over the shoulders (touching only the inside surface of the gown) and secure the ties at the back.
4. With the hands retained within the sleeves, the waist ties should be picked up and held out to the sides. In the case of a **back-tying gown**, the unscrubbed assistant will then take the ends of the waist ties and secure them at the back. The back of the gown is now no longer sterile and must not come into contact with sterile equipment, drapes and gowns.

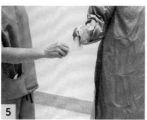

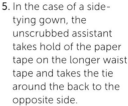

5. In the case of a side-tying gown, the unscrubbed assistant takes hold of the paper tape on the longer waist tape and takes the tie around the back to the opposite side.

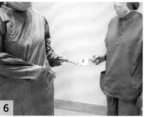

6. The scrubbed person then pulls the tape, so that the paper tape comes away.

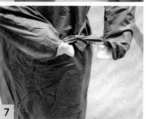

7. The gown is tied at the waist by the scrubbed person. This type of gown provides an all-round sterile field.

NOTES

Closed gloving procedure

1. Hands remain within the sleeves of the gown. The glove packet is turned so that the fingers point towards the body. (The right glove will now be on the left and *vice versa*.)
2. The glove is picked up at the rim of the cuff of the glove.
3. The hand is turned over so that the glove lies on the palm surface with fingers of the glove still pointing towards the body.
4. The rim is picked up with the opposite hand.
5. It is then pulled over the fingers and over the dorsal surface of the wrist.
6. The glove is then pulled on as the fingers are pushed forwards.

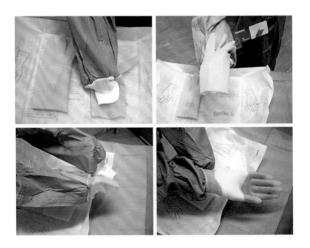

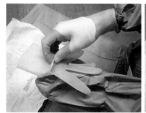

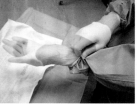

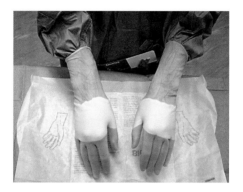

NOTES

Open gloving procedure

1. The glove pack is opened by an assistant.
2. With the left hand, the right glove is picked up by the turned-down cuff, holding only the inner surface of the glove.
3. The glove is pulled on to the right hand. Do not unfold the cuff at this stage.
4. The gloved fingers of the right hand are placed under the cuff of the left glove and pulled on to the left hand, holding only the outer surface of this glove.
5. The rim of the left glove is hooked over the thumb whilst the cuff of the gown (if worn) is adjusted.
6. The cuff of the left glove is pulled over the cuff of the gown (if worn) using the fingers of the right hand.
7. The final steps are then repeated for the right hand.

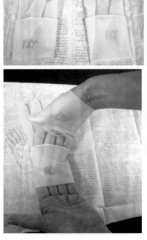
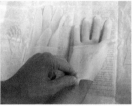
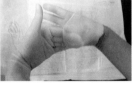

Haematology reference ranges [16]

Species	RBC count (10^{12}/l)	WBC count (10^9/l)	PCV (%)	Hb (g/dl)	MCV (fl)	MCHC (g/dl)
Dog	5.5–8.5	6–17	37–55	12–18	60–70	32–36
Cat	5–10	5.5–19.5	24–45	9–17	39–55	30–36

See also **Biochemistry reference ranges; Packed cell volume – how to perform a PCV**

NOTES

Hair and skin sampling procedures [9, 13, 16]

Handheld lens examination

Indications

- Fleas, flea dirt, lice, and *Cheyletiella*.

Equipment

- Low-power handheld magnifying lens.

Technique

Examine skin and hair with lens.

Wood's lamp

Indications

- Some strains of *Microsporum canis* fluoresce when exposed to ultraviolet light.

Equipment

- Wood's lamp (ideally double tube); gloves; protective clothing; dark room.

Technique

Allow the lamp to warm up (5–10 minutes). In a dark room, expose hairs for 3–5 minutes (some are slow to respond). 50% of *Microsporum canis* will fluoresce apple green in colour. If positive, perform hair plucking and culture on dermatophyte test medium or Sabouraud's medium, or send to outside laboratory. **Note:** Some bacteria, skin debris or certain drugs may fluoresce and give false positive results.

Coat brushing

Indications

- Fleas, lice, *Cheyletiella*, dermatophytes (ringworm).

Equipment

- Fine-toothed comb; paper for collection of material; microscope slides; liquid paraffin; pipette; coverslips; microscope.

Technique

Stand the patient over paper. Groom animal's coat with comb. Examine debris with handheld magnifying lens. Place some debris on a slide with a drop of liquid paraffin and apply a coverslip. Examine under low power microscope. Use damp cotton wool to examine suspected flea dirt (turns reddish brown at edge of dirt). Samples for an outside laboratory should go into paper packs, e.g. Dermpacks.

Mackenzie brush

Indications

- Dermatophytes or spores of dermatophytes.

Equipment

- Mackenzie brush; growth medium.

Technique

Sterile toothbrush is brushed through coat to collect hairs. Press toothbrush on to dermatophyte test medium or Sabouraud's medium for culture.

Skin scraping

Indications

- For detection of all mites, particularly those living deep in the skin.

Equipment

- Clippers and clipper blades (size 40); size 10 scalpel blade (blunt); liquid paraffin or 10% potassium hydroxide; microscope slide; glass coverslip; china-graph pen/permanent marker and microscope. ⟹

Technique

1. Put on gloves.
2. Select the area to be scraped.
3. Clip the area (if necessary) using the clippers; this will allow more accurate scraping and will remove hair that may obscure findings. Clipping is not usually necessary where surface-dwelling parasites are suspected.
4. Dip the scalpel blade into liquid paraffin or potassium hydroxide, which will act as a mounting medium and moisten the surface of the skin. This will make the detection and identification of the ectoparasites easier.
5. Hold the blade between the thumb and forefinger.
6. Stretch the skin to be scraped with the other hand and then gently scrape the area (usually a 3 cm by 3 cm area). The depth of scraping will vary according to the parasite in question, although most scraping should result in a small amount of capillary ooze.
7. Transfer the collected material from the forward surface of the blade on to a glass slide. A drop of liquid paraffin or 10% potassium hydroxide can be added to the slide.
8. Place a coverslip over the top of the sample and label the slide.
9. Set up the microscope and examine the slide using the lowest power first. Vernier scale readings can be used to record the location of parasites, although live parasites may move.
10. Slides should be viewed immediately after the sample has been collected to avoid parasites leaving the slide.
11. Once the slide has been examined and results recorded, dispose of it in a sharps container.

Ear swab collection

Indications
- For detection of *Otodectes* ear mites.

Equipment
- Gloves; appropriate swabs; pen for labelling.

Technique
1. Wear gloves.
2. Select appropriate swab (e.g. charcoal for bacteriology).
3. Ask for assistance and give instructions for the animal to be restrained.
4. Collect sufficient material for analysis by gently rotating the swab to cover all surfaces without traumatizing the ear or causing any discomfort; avoid any contamination.
5. Replace the swab into the cover tube without any further contamination and secure the lid.
6. Remove gloves and ensure correct disposal.
7. Label the swab with the location the sample was collected from (e.g. 'right ear').
8. Label the swab with the animal's name, owner's name and the date.
9. Package the swab following packaging guidelines.

Hair plucking

Indications
- Samples for fungal culture or trichograms, dermatophytes (ringworm), occasionally *Demodex*.

Equipment
- Broad-rimmed epilation forceps; slides; liquid paraffin; gloves.

Technique
Look for hairs immersed in scale and crust. Pluck single, entire hairs from the edges of lesions, using epilation. ▪▪▪➡

For in-house examination

Place hair on slide. Add liquid paraffin or stain (lactophenol cotton blue or Quink black/blue ink). Examine under microscope. Affected material including hair shaft will stain blue.

For an outside laboratory

Place hair sample in clearly labelled paper envelope.

Sticky tape preparation – 1

Indications

- Lice and *Cheyletiella*.

Equipment

- Scissors or clippers; clear sticky tape (19 mm wide); liquid paraffin; microscope slides; microscope.

Technique

Select areas of dry scaly skin and scurfy hair. Clip hair carefully, avoiding skin surface. Apply sticky surface of adhesive tape to skin and base of hairs. Add a small drop of liquid paraffin to a microscope slide. Place tape (sticky side down) on to microscope slide. Examine immediately using low power objective.

Sticky tape preparation – 2

Indications

- *Malassezia* and bacteria.

Equipment

- As above plus: Scotch tape 19 mm (other tapes unsuitable for staining); Diff-Quik® or Rapi-Diff stains; tissues; microscope; immersion oil.

Technique

Select area of greasy, erythematous skin (axillae, inguinal and interdigital regions). Clip hair carefully. Apply sticky surface of adhesive tape several times to skin. Stain sticky tape with Diff-Quik®. Attach tape, sticky side down, to microscope slide. Cover with paper tissues and exert gentle pressure to remove excess fluid. Examine immediately using X40 or X100 under oil immersion.

Impression smears

Indications

- Cytological assessment or *Demodex*.

Equipment

- Microscope slide; microscope.

Technique

Slide is pressed directly against lesion and smeared. Air-dry slide. Stain for cytology. Examine under microscope.

Fine needle aspiration

Indications

- *Demodex*, bacteria, cytology.

Equipment

- Sterile 5 ml syringe; sterile 25 G needle; microscope slides; coverslip; microscope.

Technique

Aspirate pustule or nodule contents using a sterile syringe and needle. Express contents on to slide. Smear or place coverslip on top. Examine under the microscope.

Skin biopsy

Indications

- Histopathology, dermatophytes, *Malassezia*, bacteria and occasionally mites.

Equipment

- Biopsy punch or scalpel blade and handle; sterile swabs; 10% formalin in wide-mouthed container; shiny card; sterile needle; suture material and instruments.

Technique

Clip hair carefully, avoiding skin. Collect sample, using biopsy punch or an elliptical incision. Blot off excess fluid with a sterile swab (so that it does not slip off the card). Using a sterile needle, place dermal layer in contact with shiny card. Place in 10% formalin immediately (cells deteriorate very quickly if left exposed to air). Close skin with a single suture.

NOTES

Hand hygiene

- Effective hand hygiene and disinfection should be practised between all patients.
- A handwashing procedure, such as that recommended by the World Health Organization (WHO) should be followed.
- Hands should be washed:
  - Before and after touching a patient
  - Before and after touching a patient's surroundings or any potential fomites
  - Before gloving
  - Before any clean or aseptic task
  - After any risk of exposure to contaminated fluids or tissue (even if gloves have been worn)
  - Between patients.

How to handwash?

Wash hands when visibly soiled! Otherwise, use handrub
Duration of the entire procedure: 40–60 seconds

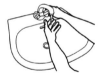

0 Wet hands with water

1 Apply enough soap to cover all hand surfaces

2 Rub hands palm to palm

3 Right palm over left dorsum with interlaced fingers and vice versa

4 Palm to palm with fingers interlaced

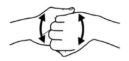

5 Backs of fingers to opposing palms with fingers interlocked

6 Rotational rubbing of left thumb clasped in right palm and vice versa

7 Rotational rubbing, backwards and forwards with clasped fingers of right hand in left palm and vice versa

8 Rinse hands with water

9 Dry hands thoroughly with a single use towel

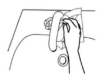

10 Use towel to turn off faucet

11 Your hands are now safe

World Health Organization (WHO) poster providing instructions on how to hand wash. (© World Health Organization 2009)

Infection control [12, 16, 20]

Infection prevention and control procedures are essential to protect patients, owners, veterinary staff and the wider community. Whilst it is impossible to completely prevent hospital-acquired infections (HAIs) from occurring, the implementation of a structured 'best practice' infection control programme can limit their occurrence.

Protocols must include:

- Hand hygiene (*see* **Hand hygiene**)
- Environmental cleaning and disinfection (*see* **Cleaning the operating theatre**)
- Fomite consideration
- Surgical asepsis and technique (including the theatre environment, patient preparation, the surgeon and theatre staff) (*see* **Gowning and gloving, Scrubbing, Theatre – maintenance of asepsis**)
- Antibiotic stewardship (*see* **PROTECT ME**)
- Wound management (*see* **Wound drain management**)
- Isolation and barrier nursing for infectious and immunosuppressed patients.

It is important to understand the various transmission routes of pathogens. Infection control and prevention depends on the disruption of the transmission of pathogens from infected animals or humans to new hosts or locations. Understanding routes of disease transmission and how they contribute to the spread of the organisms will identify effective infection control measures not only for specific diseases, but also for other pathogens transmitted by similar routes, including unanticipated infectious diseases.

Whilst it remains the responsibility of veterinary staff to prevent the spread of pathogens and disease within the practice, it is imperative that clients are also sufficiently educated on the role they have regarding biosecurity in the community and their home environment. As well as general infectious disease education, clients should be informed on zoonotic and vector-borne risks relevant to their pets, themselves, and family members.

Useful websites for further reading

BSAVA knowledge bank:
www.bsava.com/MyBSAVA/Knowledge-bank/Practice/
Practice-Pack/Module-7

The Bella Moss Foundation:
www.thebellamossfoundation.com

NOTES

Intravenous catheter management [4, 16]

- Management must be exemplary, as many critically ill patients are immunosuppressed and likely to contract infections easily.
- Hands must be washed before handling of catheters and gloves worn. Ensure aseptic handling of the catheter at all times.
- Clean any spilt blood from around the catheter with antiseptic solution, and ensure that all tapes securing catheters and dressings are clean.
- The use of impregnated dressings may be helpful in immunocompromised patients.
- Maintain catheter patency by flushing with heparinized saline (4 units of heparin per 1 ml of 0.9% saline) every 4–6 hours.
- Change peripheral catheters regularly (usually every 3–5 days), in line with instructions from the veterinary surgeon in charge. Jugular lines are rarely changed if they are functioning well.
- Inspect the skin insertion site of jugular catheters at least daily, preferably twice daily, with gloved hands. Check for signs of infection, perivascular administration of fluid, leakage of fluid from the catheter and giving set junction, or 'blowing' of the vein.
- Replace the sterile dressing daily.

NOTES

NOTES

NOTES

NOTES

Laboratory samples – packaging for external analysis[13, 16]

Labelling and paperwork

Each sample should be labelled with the owner's name, the animal's name or reference number, the type of sample collected and the date of collection (e.g. 'Fluffy Brown – Urine 24/2/12').

An appropriate submission form should accompany every sample submitted to an external laboratory. If a submission form is not available, similar information should be provided in an accompanying letter. This information ensures that the laboratory performs the appropriate test and is able to interpret the results. Forms should be placed in a plastic envelope to prevent contamination should the container break in transit.

INFORMATION REQUIRED BY EXTERNAL LABORATORIES

- Practice details and veterinary surgeon's name
- Owner's name and address
- Animal's name or reference number
- Species, breed, age and sex (M, MN, F, FN)
- Date of sampling and time of collection
- Date of dispatch of sample
- Clinical history (including presenting signs) and current treatments
- Types of samples collected (including type of preservatives used)
- Site(s) of sample collection
- Test or examination required

Postage and packaging

Samples that are not preserved, packed or posted appropriately may be damaged in transit. Damaged samples can produce inaccurate results and it is therefore extremely important to ensure that samples arrive in the best possible condition.

- Check the information supplied by the laboratory to ensure that the correct types of sample are being sent.
- Do not post samples on a Friday, as they will sit in a warm post box all weekend.

The following are rules for postage of pathological samples, and *must* be adhered to.

- The sender must ensure that the sample will not expose anyone to danger (COSHH 1988).
- A *maximum* sample of 50 ml is allowed through the post, unless by specific arrangement with Royal Mail.
- Samples must be labelled correctly with time, date, owner and animal identification, and nature of the sample (e.g. 'heparinized plasma').
- *Primary container* must be leak-proof and must be wrapped in enough absorbent material to absorb the complete sample if leakage or breakage occurs.
- The wrapped sample is then placed in a *leak-proof plastic bag*.
- This is placed in a secondary container (e.g. polypropylene clip-down container or cylindrical metal container).
- Seal the correctly completed laboratory form in a plastic bag for extra protection and place with sample.
- Place in a tertiary container (strong cardboard or grooved polystyrene box), approved by Royal Mail, and seal securely.
- *Outer packaging must be labelled conspicuously:* FRAGILE WITH CARE / PATHOLOGICAL SPECIMEN / ADDRESS OF LABORATORY / Address of sender.
- Almost all samples sent from veterinary practices to laboratories are classed as 'diagnostic substances' and outer packaging must clearly show 'Diagnostic specimen Licence no. UN3373' with diamond shaped mark.
- Ensure the sample is sent by first class post or via a courier.

If the Royal Mail's conditions are not complied with the sender is liable to prosecution.

NOTES

NOTES

Mucous membrane colour[16]

- Normal oral mucous membranes should be **pink** in colour.
- **Pale** membranes are indicative of poor perfusion; this may be seen in patients with circulatory collapse, anaemia, haemorrhage or severe vasoconstriction.
- **Red** (congested) membranes may indicate sepsis, fever, congestion, causes of extensive tissue damage or excitement.
- **Blue or purple** membranes (cyanosis) indicate severe hypoxaemia (lack of oxygen in the blood). This could be caused by respiratory difficulty and immediate action must be taken to increase the patient's oxygen saturation.
- **Yellow** membranes (icterus/jaundice) may be due to liver disease, bile flow obstruction or an increase in red blood cell destruction and circulating bilirubin.
- **Chocolate brown** membranes in dogs and cats are indicative of paracetamol poisoning. Cats are unable to metabolize paracetamol and thus toxicity can occur after the consumption of even low doses.
- **Cherry red** membranes are seen in patients suffering from carbon monoxide poisoning (e.g. following exposure to car exhaust or smoke fumes).

NOTES

Muscle condition scoring scheme — cats[21]

Muscle condition score is assessed by visualization and palpation of the spine, scapulae, skull, and wings of the ilia. Muscle loss is typically first noted in the epaxial muscles on each side of the spine; muscle loss at other sites can be more variable. Muscle condition score is graded as normal, mild loss, moderate loss, or severe loss. Note that animals can have significant muscle loss even if they are overweight (body condition score >5/9). Conversely, animals can have a low body condition score (<4/9) but have minimal muscle loss. Therefore, assessing both body condition score and muscle condition score on every animal at every visit is important. Palpation is especially important with mild muscle loss and in animals that are overweight. An example of each score is shown below.

Normal muscle mass

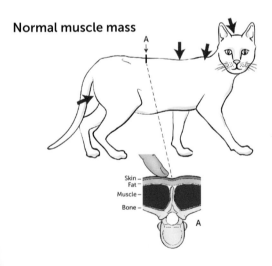

Skin
Fat
Muscle
Bone

Mild muscle loss

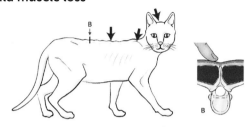

Moderate muscle loss

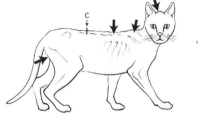

Severe muscle loss

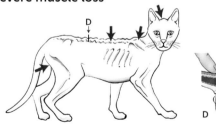

Provided courtesy of the World Small Animal Veterinary Association (WSAVA). Available at the WSAVA Global Nutrition Committee Nutritional Toolkit website: wsava.org/global-guidelines/global-nutrition-guidelines. Accessed August 2020 Copyright Tufts University, 2014

Muscle condition scoring scheme – dogs[21]

Muscle condition score is assessed by visualization and palpation of the spine, scapulae, skull, and wings of the ilia. Muscle loss is typically first noted in the epaxial muscles on each side of the spine; muscle loss at other sites can be more variable. Muscle condition score is graded as normal, mild loss, moderate loss, or severe loss. Note that animals can have significant muscle loss if they are overweight (body condition score >5/9). Conversely, animals can have a low body condition score (<4) but have minimal muscle loss. Therefore, assessing both body condition score and muscle condition score on every animal at every visit is important. Palpation is especially important when muscle loss is mild and in animals that are overweight. An example of each score is shown below.

Normal muscle mass

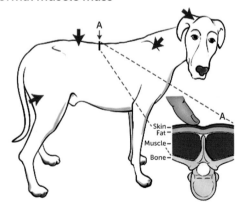

Skin
Fat
Muscle
Bone

Mild muscle loss

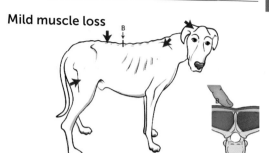

Moderate muscle loss

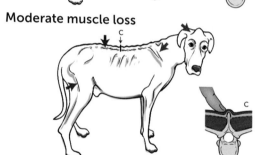

Severe muscle loss

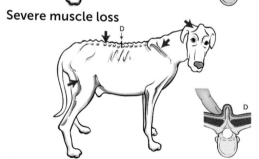

Provided courtesy of the World Small Animal Veterinary
Association (WSAVA). Available at the WSAVA Global Nutrition
Committee Nutritional Toolkit website: wsava.org/global-
guidelines/global-nutrition-guidelines. Accessed August 2020
Copyright Tufts University, 2013

NOTES

Opioids [5, 16]

Drug	Opioid receptor effects	Analgesic efficacy	Duration of action	Routes of administration	Controlled Drug status
Morphine	Mu agonist	Potent analgesic agent	2–6 hours	i.v. (dilute with saline and give slowly; bolus or CRI), i.m., s.c. epidural (use a preservative-free solution)	Schedule 2
Methadone	Mu agonist	Equipotent to morphine	4–8 hours	i.v., i.m., s.c. Not routinely given by CRI or epidural	Schedule 2
Pethidine	Mu agonist	Potent but very short-acting	1–1.5 hours	i.m., s.c. Do not give i.v.	Schedule 2
Fentanyl	Mu agonist	More potent than morphine	20–30 minutes	i.v. (CRI or bolus)	Schedule 2
Buprenorphine	Partial mu agonist	Significantly less potent than morphine	4–12 hours	i.v., i.m., s.c. (not recommended), oral, transmucosal	Schedule 3
Butorphanol	Mu antagonist/ kappa agonist	Poor analgesic but good sedation	1.5–2 hours	i.v., i.m., s.c.	Not subject to Controlled Drug Regulations
Naloxone	Antagonist	No analgesic properties (opioid reversal)	30–60 minutes	i.v.	Not subject to Controlled Drug Regulations

NOTES

Packed cell volume – how to perform a PCV[16]

Packed cell volume (PCV) (also known as the haematocrit) is the percentage of the total blood volume that is occupied by red blood cells. This quick and easy test rapidly gives information on hydration status, level of blood loss in haemorrhaging patients, or degree of anaemia.

PREPARING A PCV SAMPLE

1. Put on gloves.
2. Select a blood sample with EDTA.
3. Mix the sample gently.
4. Remove plain microhaematocrit capillary tubes from their container (1 or 2).
5. Insert a microhaematocrit tube into the sample (holding the sample tube at an angle) and fill the tube to at least three-quarters full by capillary action.
6. Place a finger over the top end of the tube or keep the tube horizontal to prevent leakage of blood.
7. Remove the tube from the sample.
8. Wipe the outside of the tube with a tissue.
9. Plug one end of the tube with soft clay sealant.
10. Place the tube into the microhaematocrit centrifuge with the clay plug against the rim.
11. Balance the centrifuge with a second tube.
12. Screw the inner safety lid down over the samples.
13. Close and lock the main lid.
14. Set at 10,000 rpm (or fast setting, depending on make of centrifuge) for 5 minutes.
15. Dispose of any used capillary tubes and other used materials as hazardous waste.

Once the microhaematocrit tube has been centrifuged the blood will have separated into three layers: red cells, buffy coat and plasma.

Ideally, the PCV should be read using a Hawksley microhaematocrit reader (see below). If one is not available a ruler can be used along with the following calculation:

PCV (%) = (height of red blood cells/total column height) x 100

Using a Hawksley PCV reader

1. Place the tube into the slot in the reader, with the sealed end downwards.
2. Align the top of the seal, i.e. the bottom of the red blood cell layer, with the zero line on the reader.

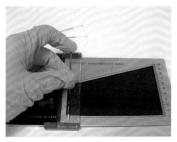

3. Move the tube holder across until the top of the plasma is lined up with the 100% line on the reader.

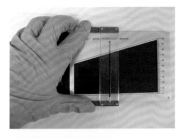

4. Move the adjustable PCV reading line to intersect the top of the RBC layer.

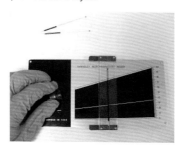

5. Record the PCV reading correctly as a percentage.

See also **Haematology reference ranges**

NOTES

Pain assessment[1, 5]

Key points

- Assume that humans and animals are similar in terms of pain perception and anticipation, and manage pain accordingly.
- At present, response to appropriate analgesia remains the best marker for accurate diagnosis of pain.
- Remember that breed, age, illness, temperament and drug administration influence behavioural responses to pain.
- Since the pain experience can alter rapidly, pain assessment must be performed frequently.
- Pain assessors should have experience in pain assessment and be familiar with the patient.
- Compare an animal's behaviour before and after the onset of pain where this is possible (i.e. pre- and postoperatively), so that improvement or deterioration can be evaluated realistically.
- Assess response to interaction with a handler in addition to simple observation in the cage.
- Assess response to gentle palpation or manipulation of the affected area.
- Look for subtle indicators of pain, particularly in sick patients. Remember that invasive procedures, trauma and medical illnesses cause pain, and may leave animals unable to demonstrate explicit pain behaviour. Certain animals may respond to pain through withdrawal.
- Develop clinic protocols for assessment of acute and chronic pain. An ideal scoring system should be relatively easy to use by all staff, with clearly defined assessment criteria, and validated in a clinical setting.
- Reassess. Re-evaluate analgesic efficacy. Re-administer analgesia appropriately as assessment requires.

Behavioural indicators of pain

- **Dog:**
  - Hyperalgesia or allodynia
  - Postures: hunching, 'praying', not resting in a normal position
  - Locomotor activity: limping and guarding, reluctance to move or lie down, stiff, partial or no weight-bearing, lameness
  - Vocalization: barking, growling, whining
  - Facial expressions: ear position, eye position
  - Attention to (or guarding of) the affected area
  - Aggression
  - Inappetence
  - Weak tail wag
  - Loss of house training.
- **Cat:**
  - As for dog, with additionally:
  - Vocalization: hissing
  - Facial expressions: furrowed brow, ears pinned back
  - Depression, no self-grooming
  - Hunched immobile stance
  - Hyperventilation
  - Sitting in back of cage or hiding under blanket
  - Pupillary dilation
  - Restlessness
  - Tachypnoea or panting.

Pain scales

- Visual analogue scale (VAS).
- Numerical rating scale (NRS).
- Simple descriptive scale (SDS).
- Composite scoring system.
- Multidimensional scoring system.

Using pain scales and scoring systems

- A patient's pain score is a composite of multidimensional factors such as behaviour, body postures, facial grimaces and (for some scales) physiological parameters that might indicate pain.
- Change in behaviour between pre- and post-painful stimulus is the most consistent indicator of the presence of pain.
- When in doubt as to whether or not a patient is in pain, the default is to administer analgesia and reassess their comfort level.

NOTES

NOTES

Pain scoring — cat [1, 5]

Pain score	Example	Psychological and behavioural	Response to palpation	Body tension
0		Animal is sleeping and cannot be evaluated		
		☐ Content and quiet when unattended ☐ Comfortable when resting ☐ Interested in or curious about surroundings	☐ Not bothered by palpation of wound or surgery site, or to palpation elsewhere	Minimal
1		☐ Signs are often subtle and not easily detected in the hospital setting: more likely to be detected by the owner(s) at home ☐ Earliest signs at home may be withdrawal from surroundings or change in normal routine ☐ In the hospital, may be content or slightly unsettled ☐ Less interested in surroundings but will look around to see what is going on	☐ May or may not react to palpation of wound or surgery site	Mild
2		☐ Decreased responsiveness, seeks solitude ☐ Quiet, loss of brightness in eyes ☐ Lays curled up or sits tucked up (all four feet under body, shoulders hunched, head held slightly lower than shoulders, tail curled tightly around body) with eyes partially or mostly closed ☐ Hair coat appears rough or fluffed ☐ May intensively groom an area that is painful or irritating ☐ Decreased appetite, not interested in food	☐ Responds aggressively or tries to escape if painful area is palpated or approached ☐ Tolerates attention, may even perk up when petted as long as painful area is avoided	Mild to moderate Reassess analgesic plan

	☐ Constantly yowling, growling, or hissing when unattended ☐ May bite or chew at wound, but unlikely to move if left alone	☐ Growls or hisses at non-painful palpation (may be experiencing allodynia, wind-up, or fearful that pain could be made worse) ☐ Reacts aggressively to palpation, adamantly pulls away to avoid any contact	Moderate Reassess analgesic plan
3			
	☐ Prostrate ☐ Potentially unresponsive to or unaware of surroundings, difficult to distract from pain ☐ Receptive to care (even mean or wild cats will be more tolerant of contact)	☐ May not respond to palpation ☐ May be rigid to avoid painful movement	Moderate to severe May be rigid to avoid painful movement Reassess analgesic plan
4			

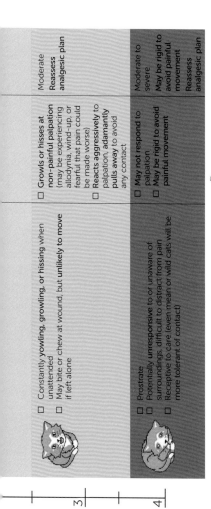

O Tender to palpation
X Warm
■ Tense

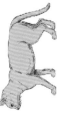

The Colorado Feline Acute Pain Scale (Reproduced with permission from Peter W. Hellyer, College of Veterinary Medicine and Biomedical Sciences, Colorado State University, USA).

Pain scoring – dog [1, 5]

Dog's name .... **Date** / / **Time**............

Hospital number ....

Procedure or condition...............................
....

In the sections below please circle the appropriate score in each list and sum these to give the total score

A. Look at dog in kennel

Is the dog

(i)
Quiet	0
Crying or whimpering	1
Groaning	2
Screaming	3

(ii)
Ignoring any wound or painful area	0
Looking at wound or painful area	1
Licking wound or painful area	2
Rubbing wound or painful area	3
Chewing wound or painful area	4

In the case of spinal, pelvic or multiple limb fractures, or where assistance is required to aid locomotion, do not carry out section **B** and proceed to **C**. Please tick if this is the case ☐ then proceed to **C**

B. Put lead on dog and lead out of the kennel

When the dog rises/walks is it?

(iii)
Normal	0
Lame	1
Slow or reluctant	2
Stiff	3
It refuses to move	4

C. If it has a wound or painful area including abdomen, apply gentle pressure 2 inches round the site

Does it? (iv)
Do nothing	0
Look round	1
Flinch	2
Growl or guard area	3
Snap	4
Cry	5

D. Overall

Is the dog? (v)
Happy and content or happy and bouncy	0
Quiet	1
Indifferent or non-responsive to surroundings	2
Nervous or anxious or fearful	3
Depressed or non-responsive to stimulation	4

Is the dog? (vi)
Comfortable	0
Unsettled	1
Restless	2
Hunched or tense	3
Rigid	4

Total score (i+ii+iii+iv+v+vi) =............

The Glasgow Composite Measure Pain Scale (short form)
(© University of Glasgow 2008; licensed to NewMetrica Ltd)

Guidance for use of the CMPS-SF

The short form composite measure pain scale (CMPS-SF) can be applied quickly and reliably in a clinical setting and has been designed as a clinical decision-making tool which was developed for dogs in acute pain. It includes 30 descriptor options within 6 behavioural categories, including mobility. Within each category, the descriptors are ranked numerically according to their associated pain severity and the person carrying out the assessment chooses the descriptor within each category which best fits the dog's behaviour/condition. It is important to carry out the assessment procedure as described on the questionnaire, following the protocol closely. The pain score is the sum of the rank scores. The maximum score for the 6 categories is 24, or 20 if mobility is impossible to assess. The total CMPS-SF score has been shown to be a useful indicator of analgesic requirement and the recommended analgesic intervention level is 6/24 or 5/20.

NOTES

Pain scoring – rabbit [1, 5, 19]

Research has demonstrated that changes in facial expression provide a means of assessing pain in rabbits.

The specific facial action units shown below comprise the Rabbit Grimace Scale. These action units increase in intensity in response to post-procedural pain and can form part of a clinical assessment alongside other validated indices of pain. The action units should only be used in awake animals. Each animal should be observed for a short period of time to avoid scoring brief changes in facial expression that are unrelated to the animal's welfare.

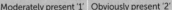

Orbital tightening

- Closing of the eyelid (narrowing of orbital area)
- A wrinkle may be visible around the eye

Not present '0'	Moderately present '1'	Obviously present '2'

Cheek flattening

- Flattening of the cheeks. When 'obviously present', cheeks have a sunken look
- The face becomes more angular and less rounded

Not present '0'	Moderately present '1'	Obviously present '2'

The Rabbit Grimace Scale. (Reproduced with permission of the NC3Rs; www.nc3rs.org.uk/grimacescales; Keating *et al.*, 2012; images provided by Dr Matthew Leach, Newcastle University)

Nostril shape

- Nostrils (nares) are drawn vertically forming a 'V' rather than 'U' shape
- Nose tip is moved down towards the chin

Not present '0'	Moderately present '1'	Obviously present '2'
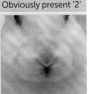		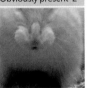

Whisker shape and position

- Whiskers are pushed away from the face to 'stand on end'
- Whiskers stiffen and lose their natural, downward curve
- Whiskers increasingly point in the same direction. When 'obviously present', whiskers move downwards

Not present '0'	Moderately present '1'	Obviously present '2'

Ear shape and position

- Ears become more tightly folded/curled (more cylindrical) in shape
- Ears rotate from facing towards the source of sound to facing towards the hindquarters
- Ears may be held closer to the back or sides of the body

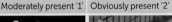

Not present '0'	Moderately present '1'	Obviously present '2'

Patient assessment — daily tasks[16]

- **Record temperature, pulse and respiration.** These are essential vital signs and it is best if the patient is calm prior to completing these assessments.
- **Record bodyweight on a weight chart.** If a 10% weight loss is identified, consideration must be given to providing nutritional support.
- **Evaluate the mental state of the patient.** Is the animal BAR, QAR, progressing or deteriorating.
- **Provide the animal with the opportunity to go outside and exercise.** 3–4 times a day is recommended for dogs.
- **Assess any wounds.** Wounds should be showing signs of healing. If there are any signs of infection, the clinical team should be informed. Dressings and bandages should be changed as required.
- **Monitor for signs of pain and discomfort.** This should be performed continually throughout the day and analgesic protocols amended if necessary.
- **Administer any prescribed medications.**
- **Provide nutrition** (unless nil by mouth). The correct amount of the right type of food should be calculated and fed to the patient. The quantity consumed should be recorded.
- **Care of intravenous cannulae.** Peripheral intravenous catheters should be flushed regularly and checked for patency. The insertion sites should be checked for any signs of infection. Cannulae should be removed and replaced if necessary.
- **Care of wound drains, cavity drains and feeding tubes.** Insertion sites should be checked at least twice daily and bandaged when required. Drained fluid should be measured and the volume recorded.
- **Physiotherapy** – should be performed on recumbent or inactive patients, usually 2–4 times a day.

Patient assessment – routine parameters [4]

Body system/ assessment	Parameter	Interval
Cardiovascular	Pulse rate and quality Mucous membranes Capillary refill time Arterial blood pressure Central venous pressure (if central catheter present)	Every 1–6 h
Respiratory	Respiratory rate and effort Oxygen saturation (pulse oximeter)	Every 1–6 h
Demeanour	Patient appearance and behaviour	Every 2–6 h
Temperature		Every 2–12 h
Urination assessment	Walk, check tray, check bladder and drain urinary collection bag Calculate ml/kg/h and specific gravity when obtainable	Every 2–4 h
Wounds/ dressings/ intravenous catheters	Tension, swelling and discharge	Every 4–12 h
Intravenous catheters	Flush	Every 4 h
Arterial catheters	Flush	Every 1 h
Recumbent patients	Ensure patient is turned	At least every 4 h

Physiotherapy [1, 13]

Positional physiotherapy

1. Encourage the patient to stand at regular intervals.
2. Support the patient in sternal recumbency with sandbags, cushions or rolled-up towels.
3. Maintain each position for 10–15 minutes, 3–4 times daily.
4. Between treatment sessions, turn laterally recumbent patients on a regular basis (every 2–4 hours throughout the day and night).

Local hypothermia

5–10 minutes every 4–6 hours

Physiological effects	Results
↓ Tissue temperature, vasoconstriction, ↓ nerve conduction, relaxation of skeletal muscle	Analgesia, ↓ oedema, ↓ bruising

Superficial hyperthermia

10–20 minutes, 4–6 times a day

Physiological effects	Results
↑ Tissue temperature, vasodilation, ↑ local circulation, ↑ metabolic rate	Relief of muscle tension, analgesia, ↓ oedema

Massage

10–20 minutes, 2–3 times per day

Physiological effects	Results
Assisted venous return to the heart, ↑ lymphatic flow, ↑ muscular motion, ↑ tissue perfusion, maintained and improved peripheral circulation	↓ Oedema, ↓ muscle tension and spasm, temporary analgesia, ↑ muscle tone, ↑ movement through stretching of adhesions, ↓ heart rate

Passive exercise

10–20 minutes, 2–3 times a day following massage

Physiological effects	Results
Stretched adhesions, maintained or improved blood and lymphatic flow, stimulated sensory nerves	↑ range of movement, prevention or improvement of contractures, improved microcirculation to muscles and joints, improvement of stiffness

1. The patient should be comfortable, supported in lateral recumbency with the affected limb uppermost. Sandbags can be used to give additional support.
2. Use one hand to stabilize the limb above or below the joint during manipulation.
3. Use the other hand for manipulation of the joint.
4. Manipulate the distal joints of the limb first, i.e. put each toe through its full range of movement.
5. Then, working up the limb, put each joint through its full range of movement as far as the hip or shoulder.
6. Move the whole limb passively in a normal ambulatory fashion.
7. When the movement at a joint is restricted, gentle overpressure can be used at the end of the range of movement.
8. As treatment progresses, range of movement at the restricted joint improves slowly.

The aim is to move each joint individually through its full range. In recumbent patients the uppermost limbs are manipulated first. The patient can then be turned and the process repeated on the other limbs.

Active movement

Treatment sessions last from a few seconds, proceeding up to 10 minutes as the patient gains strength.

Physiological effects	Results
↑ Blood supply and lymphatic drainage, ↑ muscular tone	Gradual build-up of muscular tone and strength, improved balance and coordination, patient comfort and stimulation

PROTECT ME [17]

Antibiotic use imposes a powerful selection pressure on bacteria and is the primary driver of antibiotic resistance (AMR). Eliminating unnecessary use in people and animals is, therefore, essential to safeguard this invaluable resource. PROTECT ME is a joint initiative on the responsible use of antibiotics by SAMSoc (the Small Animal Medicine Society) and the BSAVA.

PROTECT ME

P rescribe only when necessary
- Consider non-bacterial disease (e.g. viral infection, nutritional imbalance, metabolic disorders)
- Some bacterial diseases will self-resolve without antibiotics
- Offer a non-prescription form
- Perioperative antibiotics are not a substitute for surgical asepsis

R eplace with non-antibiotic treatments
- Lavage and debridement of infected material, fluid therapy, dietary management, cough suppressants and measures to address underlying conditions may negate the need for antibiotics
- Use topical preparations (ideally antiseptics) where possible to reduce selection pressure on intestinal flora (the microbiome)

O ptimise dosage protocols
- Use the shortest effective course and avoid underdosing
- Treat until clinical resolution

T reat effectively
- Consider which bacteria are likely to be involved
- Consider drug penetration of the target site (e.g. for prostatitis, osteomyelitis)
- Consider pharmacokinetics and drug interactions with concurrent medication
- Provide instructions, including demonstrations, on how to administer prescribed antibiotics

E mploy narrow spectrum
- Use narrow-spectrum, rather than broad-spectrum, antibiotics to minimize resistance
- Avoid antibiotic combination therapy
- Use culture results to support de-escalation (switch to a narrower spectrum antibiotic)

C onduct cytology and culture
- Use cytology to demonstrate bacterial involvement **and** an inflammatory response consistent with infection (e.g. intracellular bacteria)
- Collect a sample for culture **before** starting antibiotic therapy wherever possible
- Culture is essential when using prolonged (>1 week) treatment courses, where there are risk factors for resistance (e.g. healthcare associated infections, antibiotic treatment in the prior 60 days or multiple prior courses/repeated antibiotic use) and in life-threatening situations

T ailor your practice policy
- Discuss your practice's first-line antibiotic choice for each condition with your colleagues and ensure that your protocols are clear, including when the approach is **to not prescribe an antibiotic**
- Evaluate practice biosecurity and hand hygiene protocols
- Practice preventative medicine (vaccination, parasite prevention)

M onitor
- Monitor for preventable infections (e.g. surgical site infections) and alter practice protocols if needed
- Audit your own antibiotic use, particularly of EMA **Restrict** category antibiotics (fluoroquinolones/3rd generation cephalosporins), e.g. using RCVS Knowledge Audit tool

E ducate others
- Promote awareness of AMR among staff and clients
  Encourage return of leftover antibiotics for safe disposal

NOTES

Radiographic film faults [13, 16,]

Manual radiography faults

Fault	Causes
Background too light	Probably underdeveloped Possibly underexposed (exposure too low) Low line voltage
Poorly penetrated 'silhouette' image	Underexposed or underdeveloped
Penetrated image with a thin background	Overexposed and underdeveloped (Underdevelopment leads to overexposure)
Background correct but image too dark	Overexposed (exposure factors too high) Fogged (chemicals, light, wrong safelight filter or bulb) White light leakage into darkroom or cassette Old film or film exposed to scatter/chemicals, pressure Overdeveloped
Blurred image	Movement of the patient, tube head or cassette during exposure Poor screen–film contact Incorrect screen Scatter Film fogging
Film discoloured after storage	Poorly washed or poorly fixed film
White marks on the film	Dirt or scratch on the screen Scratch on film before exposure or after processing Splash of fixer on to film or greasy fingerprints before developing
Black marks on the film	Scratch on film between exposure and processing Splash of developer before processing Water splash after developing Bending or pressure after exposure ('crimp marks')
High contrast	Low kV technique used ⟹

Fault	Causes
Low contrast	High kV Scatter (no grid used) Poor processing (e.g. exhausted developer)
Uneven processing	Poorly mixed chemicals Films touching during processing Poor agitation of films during processing
Black spots or lightning-like lines	Static electricity

Digital radiography faults

Fault	Causes
Grainy or 'noisy' appearance (quantum mottle)	Underexposure
Areas of low radiographic density are black/not discernible	Extreme overexposure
Small white marks on the image	Dirt on the phosphor
Thin linear white marks	Dirt on the rollers or light guide in the digitizer
Fading of the image	Delayed scanning of the cassettes (>24 hours)
Parts of the image are not displayed or are blacked out	Inadequate collimation in the region of interest (can be fixed during post-processing by reapplying the collimation)
Radiolucent-like appearance or 'halo' around areas with large differences in radiopacity (e.g. orthopaedic implants)	Überschwinger artefact (can be mistaken for loosening of an implant or low-grade infection)
Alternating light and dark bands across the image	Moiré artefact (stationary grid has been used, or grid aligned with the readout of the computed radiography cassette)

Radiographic positioning [3, 8, 11, 13]

Lateral view of the skull

Beam centring

Lateral canthus of eye.

Positioning and collimation

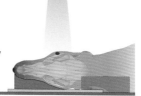

Place into lateral recumbency with affected side next to cassette. Place a foam wedge under the ramus of the mandible to stop rotation. The nasal septum should be parallel to the cassette. Place another wedge under the cranioventral cervical region; pull the front limbs caudally. Collimate to include the tip of the nose to the base of the skull.

Dorsoventral view of the skull

Beam centring

Lateral canthus of eye, over high point of cranium.

Positioning and collimation

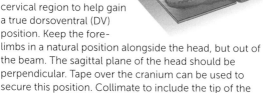

Place into sternal recumbency with the head resting on the cassette. A sandbag should be placed gently over the cervical region to help gain a true dorsoventral (DV) position. Keep the fore-limbs in a natural position alongside the head, but out of the beam. The sagittal plane of the head should be perpendicular. Tape over the cranium can be used to secure this position. Collimate to include the tip of the nose to the base of the skull.

⊪➡

Ventrodorsal view of the skull

Beam centring

Lateral canthus of eye, midline mandibular rami.

Positioning and collimation

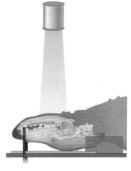

Place into dorsal recumbency. A trough or sandbags can be used to keep animal in position. The front limbs are extended caudally and secured. A foam pad should be placed under the mid-cervical region to gain proper positioning of the skull on the cassette. The nose must remain parallel to the cassette, and the skull must be balanced in a true ventrodorsal (VD) position. Place a small pad under the cranium to prevent rotation, if needed. Collimate to include the tip of the nose to the base of skull.

Lateral oblique view of the tympanic bullae

Beam centring

Over centre of tympanic bullae.

Positioning and collimation

Place into lateral recumbency with unaffected tympanic bulla toward the cassette. The forelimbs are extended slightly caudally. The skull should lie naturally at 8–12° rotation from true lateral. This causes the tympanic bullae to lie separately, allowing visualization of a single bulla. This view can also be used to examine an oblique projection of the temporomandibular joints.

Rostrocaudal view of the frontal sinuses

Beam centring

Through centre of frontal sinuses between eyes.

Positioning and collimation

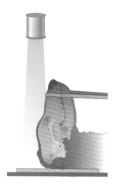

Place into dorsal recumbency with the nose pointing upwards. Pull forelimbs caudally alongside the body. Nose is positioned perpendicular to cassette. Apply a tie around the nose to stabilize. A tongue clamp may also be used to help secure, if needed. Collimate to include the entire forehead of the patient.

Dorsoventral intraoral view of the maxilla

Beam centring

Over site of interest.

Positioning and collimation

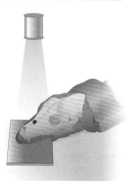

Place into sternal recumbency with the head kept in line with the spine. Place a non-screen film into the mouth, and advance caudally between the lips. The X-ray tube should be elevated to compensate for the reduction in source-to-image distance.

Ventrodorsal intraoral view of the mandible

Beam centring
Over site of interest.

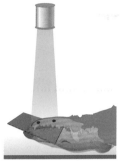

Positioning and collimation
Place into dorsal recumbency. Extend the head cranially. Place a non-screen film into the mouth with the corner edge of the film introduced first. Advance until the lips allow no further. Pull the tongue cranially to eliminate uneven density over the mandibular area. Because the source-to-image distance is reduced (as the film is elevated from the table), the X-ray tube should be raised to compensate.

Ventrodorsal open-mouth view of the nasal cavity

Beam centring
Through level of third upper premolar. To centre on nasal cavity.

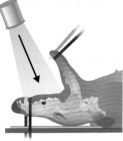

Positioning and collimation
Place into dorsal recumbency, extending forelimbs caudally alongside the body. Keep the maxilla parallel to the cassette and secure with a tie or tape. Tie the endotracheal tube to the mandible. Apply a tie around the mandible and pull in a caudal direction to open the mouth (a tongue clamp may also be used, also being secured caudally). Angle the tube head to 10–15°, to direct into the mouth. Collimate to include the entire maxilla from the tip of the nose to the pharyngeal region.

Open-mouth lateral oblique view of the lower dental arcade

Beam centring
Over site of interest.

Positioning and collimation

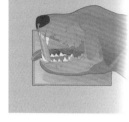

Place into lateral recumbency with affected mandible next to the cassette. Place a radiolucent gag into the mouth, to separate the upper and lower jaws. Rotate the cranium approximately 20° away from the tabletop and maintain this position with a foam wedge.

Open-mouth ventrodorsal oblique view of the upper dental arcade

Beam centring
Over third premolar.

Positioning and collimation

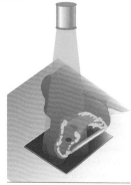

Place the patient halfway on to its back with the maxillary arcade of interest closest to the cassette. Rotate the head approx. 45° to the cassette, and stabilize on a foam wedge. The rotation prevents superimposition. Maintain the mouth open with use of a radiolucent mouth gag or by securing the mandible back, with the tongue being pulled back by a tongue depressor.

⟩⟩⟩▶

Ventrodorsal oblique view of the temporomandibular joint (TMJ)

Beam centring
Over centre of TMJ.

Positioning and collimation
Place in lateral recumbency with affected side next to the cassette. Rotate the cranium 20° towards the cassette. Place a sponge wedge under the mandible to secure the skull into position. This rotation will help prevent super-imposition. This view can be taken with or without the mouth open. Collimate to include the temporomandibular joint.

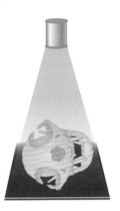

Rostrocaudal open-mouth view of the tympanic bullae

Beam centring
At level of commissure of lips.

Positioning and collimation
Place into dorsal recumbency with nose pointing upwards and forelimbs pulled caudally, along the body. Secure the

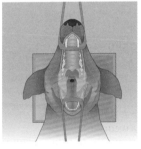

mouth open with ties and tongue clamp, and pull caudally. Pull the nose 5–10° cranially, pulling the mandible caudally. The bullae should be projected free from the mandible and the hard palate of the maxilla. Collimate to include the entire nasopharyngeal region of the skull.

Rostrocaudal view of the cranium

Beam centring
Midpoint between eyes.

Positioning and collimation
Place into dorsal recumbency with the nose pointing upwards and forelimbs pulled caudally alongside the body. Angle the nose slightly caudally (approx. 10–15°). A tie around the nose (± tongue clamp) may be used to secure this position. Collimate to include the entire cranium. *Warning: ensure endotracheal tube does not kink.*

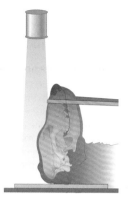

Lateral view of the pharynx

Beam centring
Over pharynx.

Positioning and collimation
Place into lateral recumbency. Extend forelimbs caudally. Extend head and neck cranially. Place a wedge under the

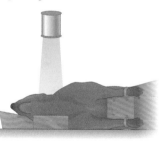

mandible, to help prevent rotation. The upper respiratory tract passages act as a negative contrast agent allowing the structures of the pharynx to be visible. Collimate to include the entire area of the neck between the lateral canthus of the eye and the 3rd cervical vertebral body.

〉〉〉➡

The vertebral column

Beam centring
Over site of interest.

Positioning and collimation
Position the vertebral column parallel to the X-ray table and perpendicular to the X-ray beam. Use radiolucent positioning aids to prevent sagging in the sagittal plane, and support the skull, sternum and limbs to limit rotation in the tranverse plane. To avoid distortion at the outer margin of the image, collimate to only include parts of the vertebral column, usually three or four vertebrae for the cervical, thoracic and lumbar regions at a time, with some images centred on the border area between two regions.

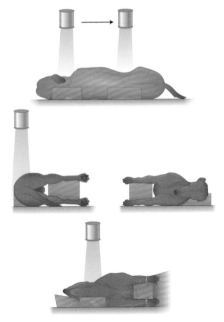

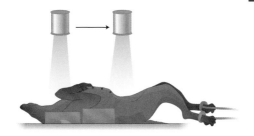

Flexed lateral view of the cervical spine

Beam centring

C3–4 intervertebral space.

Positioning and collimation

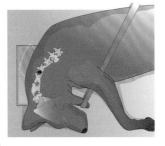

Place into lateral recumbency. Pull forelimbs in a caudal direction. Place a tie around the mandible and pull caudally (between the forelimbs). A small wedge should be placed along the spine, to prevent rotation. Collimate to include base of skull and first few thoracic vertebrae.

Warning: care must be taken not to bend the endotracheal tube causing a blockage, or further traumatize the spine (i.e. atlanto-axial subluxation).

Extended lateral view of the cervical spine

Beam centring

Intervertebral space of C4 and C5.

Positioning and collimation

Place into lateral recumbency. Extend the head and neck, pull forelimbs caudally. Push the head in a cranial direction, and secure with a tie. Place a foam wedge under the mandible to prevent rotation. Another wedge under the mid-cervical region may be necessary. Collimate to include base of the skull, entire cervical spine and first few thoracic vertebrae. Larger patients (>27 kg) may require two views: (i) base of skull to C4, (centring on C2–3); (ii) C4 to T1 (centring on C5–6).

Ventrodorsal view of the cervical spine

Beam centring

Over C4–5 intervertebral space.

Positioning and collimation

Place into dorsal recumbency. Extend the head cranially and pull forelimbs cranially along the body. Place a small wedge under the mid-cervical region to eliminate any distortion. Collimate to include the base of the skull, entire cervical spine and the first few thoracic vertebrae. Larger patients (>27 kg) may require two views: (i) base of skull to C4 (centring on C2–3); (ii) C4 to T1 (centring on C5–6).

Lateral view of the thoracic spine

Beam centring

Over 7th thoracic vertebral body.

Positioning and collimation

Place into lateral recumbency. Extend forelimbs cranially and hindlimbs caudally. Place a wedge under the sternum so that the sternum is at the same height as the thoracic vertebrae. Collimate to include the area from the 7th cervical vertebral body to the 1st lumbar vertebral body.

Ventrodorsal view of the thoracic spine

Beam centring

Over level of caudal border of scapula.

Positioning and collimation

Place into dorsal recumbency. Extend forelimbs cranially. Allow hindlimbs to lie naturally. The sternum should superimpose the thoracic spine; a trough may be required. Collimate to include all the thoracic vertebrae from C7 to L1.

Lateral view of the thoracolumbar spine

Beam centring

Over thoracolumbar junction.

Positioning and collimation

Place into lateral recumbency. Extend forelimbs cranially and hindlimbs caudally. Place a wedge under the sternum to bring it level with the spine. Collimate to include the entire thoracolumbar spine.

Ventrodorsal view of the thoracolumbar spine

Beam centring

Over thoracolumbar junction.

Positioning and collimation

Place into dorsal recumbency. Extend forelimbs cranially. Hindlimbs can lie in their natural position. Superimpose the sternum with the thoracic vertebrae; a trough can be used. Collimate to include all the thoracic and lumbar vertebrae.

⟫➡

Lateral view of the lumbar spine

Beam centring

Over level of 4th lumbar vertebral body.

Positioning and collimation

Place into lateral recumbency. Extend the forelimbs cranially and hindlimbs caudally. Place foam wedges under the sternum, mid-lumbar region and between the hind-limbs to prevent rotation. Collimate to include the 13th thoracic vertebral body to the 1st sacral vertebral body.

Ventrodorsal view of the lumbar spine

Beam centring

Over 4th lumbar vertebral body.

Positioning and collimation

Place into dorsal recumbency with forelimbs extended cranially. Allow hindlimbs to lie in natural position; wedges may be placed under the stifles and use a trough to stabilize. Collimate to include the entire lumbar spine from the 13th thoracic vertebral body to the 1st sacral vertebral body.

Lateral view of the thorax

Beam centring

Over caudal border of scapula.

Positioning and collimation

Place into right lateral recumbency – this provides the most accurate view of the cardiac silhouette. If lung metastases are suspected, both right and left views should be obtained for any subtle changes. Extend forelimbs cranially; this helps reduce superimposition of the triceps and humeri over the cranial aspect of the thorax. Extend hindlimbs slightly caudally. Extend the head slightly. Place a wedge under the mandible and thorax, and between the hindlimbs, to prevent rotation. Collimate to include the entire thoracic cavity from the line of the manubrium sterni caudally to the 1st lumbar vertebral body. Exposure is taken at full inspiration.

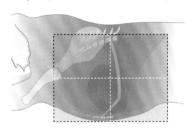

Dorsoventral view of the thorax

Beam centring
Over caudal border of scapula.

Positioning and collimation
A DV view is best for evaluation of the heart, because the heart is nearer the sternum and it sits in its normal position. This position is difficult for deep-chested breeds; use plenty of wedges and positioning aids; if unable to obtain, a VD view will have to be taken. Place into sternal recumbency. Superimpose the spine over the sternum. Extend forelimbs slightly cranially to keep elbows out of view. Hindlimbs are as normal (difficult for hip dysplastic dogs). Lower the head and place between the two forelimbs. Collimate to include the entire thorax, including all ribs. The exposure should be taken at full inspiration, to allow complete visualization of the lung tissue.

⫸

Ventrodorsal view of the thorax

Beam centring

Over caudal border of scapula.

Positioning and collimation

This view allows full visualization of the lung fields, providing better views of the accessory lung lobe and caudal mediastinum. Place into dorsal recumbency. Extend forelimbs cranially. Hindlimbs stay as normal. Superimpose the sternum with the spine. Use of a trough may help secure the position. Exposure is taken at full inspiration. *This view is contraindicated in patients with respiratory problems.*

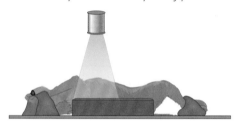

Mediolateral view of the shoulder

Beam centring

To shoulder joint.

Positioning and collimation

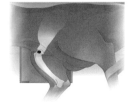

Affected limb lowermost, patient in lateral recumbency. Leg is extended cranial and ventral to sternum to prevent superimposition. Other leg is pulled in a caudodorsal direction. The neck is extended dorsally. Sternum is rotated slightly. Collimate to include the distal third of the scapula and the proximal third of the humerus.

Caudocranial view of the shoulder

Beam centring
To shoulder joint.

Positioning and collimation
Place in dorsal recumbency with both forelimbs extended cranially until parallel with cassette. *Caution: do not rotate humerus.* Collimate mid-two-thirds along scapula.

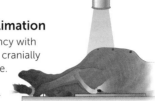

Caudocranial view of the scapula

Beam centring
Middle of scapula.

Positioning and collimation
Place in dorsal recumbency with both forelimbs extended cranially. Sternum rotated away from the scapula (approx. 10–20°). This avoids superimposing ribs. Should be a clear, unobstructed view. Collimate proximal humerus to 11th rib.

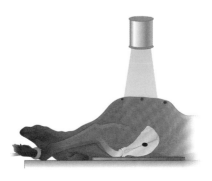

Lateral view of the humerus

Beam centring

Centre of humerus.

Positioning and collimation

Place in lateral recumbency with affected limb lowermost. Extend in cranioventral direction with the opposite limb drawn in a caudodorsal direction. Head and neck should be extended dorsally. Collimate mid-radius/ulna to distal end of scapula.

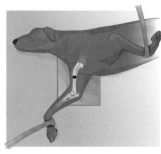

Mediolateral view of the elbow

Beam centring

Over elbow joint.

Positioning and collimation

Place in lateral recumbency with affected limb lowermost. Slightly extend the head and neck in a dorsal direction and the unaffected limb in a caudodorsal direction. Place foam wedge under the metacarpal region to maintain a true lateral view of the elbow. Collimate to include one third of the long bones either side of the joint.

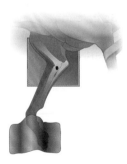

Flexed mediolateral view of the elbow

Beam centring
Middle of elbow.

Positioning and collimation

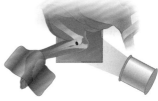

Place in lateral recumbency with affected limb lowermost. Carpus is pulled toward the neck region, flexing the elbow. Care should be taken to keep elbow in true lateral position during flexion. By keeping the carpus lateral, the elbow should also remain in a true lateral position. Collimate to include one third of the long bones either side of the joint.

Craniocaudal view of the elbow

Beam centring
Over elbow joint.

Positioning and collimation

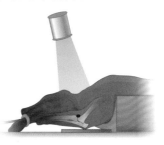

Place in sternal recumbency with the affected limb extended cranially. Elevate patient's head and position away from affected side. Exact view will provide the olecranon between the medial and lateral humeral epicondyles. Place foam pad under point of elbow to prevent rolling or rotation. Collimate to include the lateral skin edges and one third of the long bones either side of the joint.

⑄⯈

Mediolateral view of the radius and ulna

Beam centring

Middle of radius and ulna.

Positioning and collimation

Place in lateral recumbency with affected limb centred on cassette. The

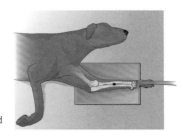

opposite limb is drawn caudally out of the way. Collimate to include the elbow and carpal joints.

Craniocaudal view of the radius and ulna

Beam centring

Middle of radius and ulna.

Positioning and collimation

Place in sternal recumbency with affected limb extended cranially. Elevate head and position away from affected side. Olecranon should be placed between the humeral condyles. Collimate to include the elbow and the carpus.

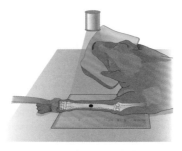

Mediolateral view of the carpus

Beam centring

Over distal row of carpal bones.

Positioning and collimation

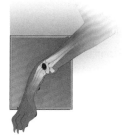

Place in lateral recumbency with affected limb in centre of cassette. Place foam wedge under elbow to prevent carpus moving away from cassette. Other leg is pulled caudally out of the way. Flexed lateral can be obtained in this position also. Collimate to include distal radius/ulna, whole of carpus and proximal end of metacarpals.

Dorsopalmar view of the carpus

Beam centring

Middle of distal row of carpal bones.

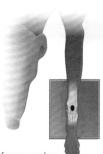

Positioning and collimation

Place in sternal recumbency with affected limb extended cranially. Carpus is flat against cassette. Place foam wedge under elbow. Oblique views are obtained with 45° angle of the dorsopalmar view to provide dorsopalmar mediolateral (DPaML) and dorsopalmar lateromedial (DPaLM) views. Stress views are with the carpus in dorsopalmar position, with radius and ulna firmly held in place. Paw is pushed medially or laterally with a ruler or a wooden paddle. Do not apply *too* much stress. Collimate to include entire carpus with two-thirds of the metacarpals and the distal end of the radius/ulna. ⅲ➡

Lateral view of the abdomen

Beam centring

Over caudal aspect of 13th rib (for feline, measure 2–3 fingerbreadths caudally).

Positioning and collimation

Place into right lateral recumbency. The right view facilitates longitudinal separation of the kidneys. Extend the hindlimbs caudally to prevent superimposition of the femoral muscles over the caudal portion of the abdomen. Place a pad between the femurs to prevent rotation of the pelvis and caudal abdomen. A pad should also be placed under the sternum, to keep sternum at the same level as the spine. Collimate to include the diaphragm caudally to the femoral head. Take the exposure at the time of expiration so that the diaphragm is displaced cranially.

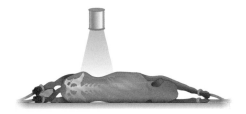

Ventrodorsal view of the abdomen

Beam centring

Over caudal aspect of 13th rib (for feline, measure 2–3 fingerbreadths caudally).

Positioning and collimation

Place into dorsal recumbency. Use a trough or sandbags for positioning. Collimate to include the diaphragm cranially, greater trochanters and lateral skin edges. Larger patients may require two views: one of the cranial abdomen and one of the caudal abdomen. Take exposure during the expiratory phase so that the diaphragm is in a cranial position and not placing any compression on the abdominal contents.

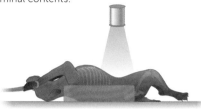

Lateral view of the pelvis

Beam centring
Over greater trochanter.

Positioning and collimation
Place into lateral recumbency with the side of interest closest to the cassette. Place foam wedge between patient's stifle joints to keep the femurs parallel to the cassette and to prevent rotation. The limb closest to the cassette should be pulled cranially, so that the femurs can be distinguished. Collimate to include entire pelvis and a portion of the lumbar spine and the femurs. Ensure the pelvis is centred to the middle of the cassette.

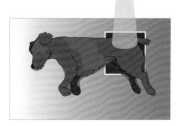

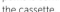

Ventrodorsal view of the pelvis – frog leg projection

Beam centring

Over level of pubis and acetabulum.

Positioning and collimation

The 'frog leg' view is suitable if pelvic trauma is suspected. Minimal stress and tension are placed on the pelvis and joints. Patient is in dorsal recumbency, placed in a trough. The femurs should be at a 45° angle; it is important for the femurs to be positioned identically to maintain symmetry.

Ventrodorsal view of the pelvis – extended projection

Beam centring

Over level of pubis and acetabulum.

Positioning and collimation

Standard evaluation for hip dysplasia. Position as for frog leg except that the hindlimbs are extended caudally, with the femurs straight and parallel to each other. Secure the stifles with Velcro or ties, and secure

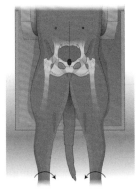

metatarsals with sandbags. The following criteria must be met:

- Femurs are parallel
- Both patellas are centred between the femoral condyles
- Pelvis is without rotation; obturator foramens, hip joints, hemipelvis and sacroiliac joints appear as a mirror image
- Tail is secured with tape between the femurs
- Collimate to include pelvis, femurs and stifle joints.

Mediolateral view of the femur

Beam centring

Middle of femur.

Positioning and collimation

Place into lateral recumbency with the affected limb closest to the cassette. Opposite limb is abducted and rotated out of the line of the X-ray beam. Place foam pad under the proximal tibia to alleviate any rotation of the femur. Collimate to include hip joint, femur and stifle joint.

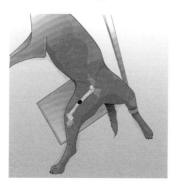

⠿➡

Craniocaudal view of the femur

Beam centring
Middle of femur.

Positioning and collimation

Place into dorsal recumbency with limb of interest extended caudally. Slight abduction of

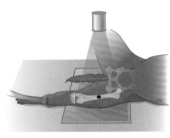

affected limb will eliminate superimposition of the proximal femur over the tuber ischium. The opposite limb is flexed and rotated laterally to facilitate abduction. The patella should be between the two femoral condyles. Collimate to include hip joint, femur and stifle joint.

Mediolateral view of the stifle

Beam centring
Over stifle joint.

Positioning and collimation

Place into lateral recumbency with the affected joint next to the cassette. The opposite limb is flexed and abducted from the line of the X-ray beam. The stifle joint should

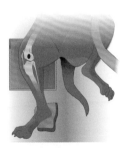

be in a natural, slightly flexed position. Place pad under the tarsus so that the tibia is parallel to cassette. Elevation of the tibia will ensure superimposition of the two femoral condyles and facilitate a true lateral view. Collimate to include the distal third of the femur and the proximal third of the tibia.

Caudocranial view of the stifle

Beam centring

Over stifle joint, distal end of the femur.

Positioning and collimation

Place into sternal recumbency with affected limb in maximum extension. Opposite limb is flexed and elevated with foam wedge. This will control the lateral rotation of the stifle joint. The

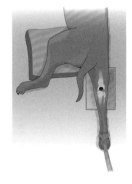

patella should be centred between the femoral condyles (which can be palpated). Collimate to include the distal third of the femur and the proximal third of the tibia.

Lateral view of the tibia and fibula

Beam centring

Middle of the tibia and fibula.

Positioning and collimation

Place into lateral recumbency with the affected limb placed on the cassette. The stifle should be flexed slightly and maintained in a true

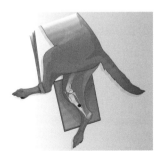

lateral position. A sponge wedge can be placed under the metatarsus to eliminate any rotation of the tibia. The opposite limb is pulled cranially or caudally so that it is out of the line of the X-ray beam. Collimate to include stifle joint, tibia and fibula, and tarsal joint.

⫸

Caudocranial view of the tibia and fibula

Beam centring

Middle of the tibia and fibula.

Positioning and collimation

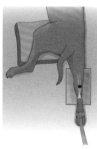

Place into sternal recumbency with the affected limb extended caudally. Support the body with foam blocks placed beneath the caudal abdomen and pelvic region. Elevating the hind end will minimize the weight placed on the stifle joint extended caudally and will facilitate positioning. The tibia/fibula should be in a true caudocranial position so that the patella is placed between the two femoral condyles. Opposite limb is flexed and placed on a pad to control rotation of the affected limb. Secure tail out of the X-ray beam. Collimate to include the stifle joint, tibia and fibula, and tarsal joint.

Mediolateral view of the tarsus

Beam centring

Middle of tarsus.

Positioning and collimation

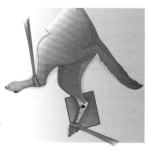

Place into lateral recumbency with affected limb next to cassette. Tarsus is placed in a natural slightly flexed position. The opposite limb should be pulled cranially out of line of the X-ray beam. Collimate to include the distal third of the tibia and the distal metatarsal bones.

Plantarodorsal view of the tarsus

Beam centring
Middle of the tarsal joint.

Positioning and collimation
Place into sternal recumbency
with the affected limb
extended as for the caudocranial view of the tibia/fibula.
Place foam blocks under the
caudal abdomen and pelvic
region to prevent tarsal

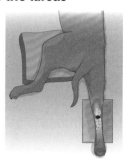

rotation. Foam blocks should also be placed under the
stifle joint to achieve maximum extension of the tarsus. If
stifle is in true caudocranial position, the tarsus will
naturally follow in a true plantarodorsal position. Collimate
to include the distal third of the tibia and the distal
metatarsal bones.

Lateral view of the phalangeal isolation

Beam centring
Centre of digit.

Positioning and collimation
Place in lateral recumbency with
affected side adjacent to cassette.
Place a foam pad under the elbow
to alleviate rotation. Superimposition is a problem here: if
one digit is to be examined, isolate
from the other digits by taping it

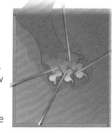

cranially in a fixed position; a further band of tape can be
used to hold the remaining digits back. Collimate distal
ulna/radius and entire paw.

Radiographic positioning — advanced [2, 4, 11]

Feline tympanic bulla

View

- Rostral 10° ventral–caudodorsal oblique (R10°V–CdDO) view

Beam centring

Centre in the midline over the pharynx, just caudal to the ramus of the mandible.

Positioning and collimation

Place the cat in dorsal recumbency supported in a trough. Secure forelimbs caudally with sandbags. Flex the head so that the hard palate is positioned 10° beyond the vertical and support in position using a foam wedge. Collimate to include the right and left skin edges to ensure the external ear canals are visible.

Comments

This view enables visualization of the tympanic bullae whilst keeping the mouth closed. It is a useful alternative to the open-mouth rostrocaudal view, especially in cats. It is important to make sure the head and body are kept in a straight line. Make sure the anaesthetic circuit is supported adequately while performing this view.

NOTES

Temporomandibular joint (TMJ)

Views

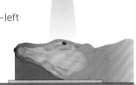

- Left lateral 20° rostral–right lateral caudal oblique (Lt20°R–RtCdO) (closed mouth) view
- Right lateral 20° rostral–left lateral caudal oblique (Rt20°R–LtCdO) (closed mouth) view

Beam centring

Centre on the caudo-ventral border of the uppermost zygomatic arch at the level of the external ear canal.

Positioning and collimation

Place the patient in lateral recumbency with the side under examination closer to the cassette. Place head in true lateral recumbency, with the hard palate positioned perpendicular to the cassette. Elevate the nose between 10° and 30° to the cassette with a triangular foam wedge:

- Dolichocephalic breeds – 10°
- Mesaticephalic breeds – 15°
- Brachycephalic breeds – 20–30°

Collimate to include the area of interest.

Comments

This view allows the TMJ to be visualized without superimposition of other structures. By raising the patient's nose, the TMJ adjacent to the cassette is highlighted rostrally and should be labelled L or R as appropriate. When investigating jaw-locking or TMJ pain, these views should be repeated with the mouth open.

▥▶

Limbs

Carpus (1)

View

- Dorsopalmar laterally and medially stressed views

Beam centring

Centre in the midline at the level of the antebrachiocarpal joint.

Positioning and collimation

Place the patient in sternal recumbency with the head supported on a foam pad to reduce rotation. Extend the forelimb under investigation cranially and secure it, using foam wedges and sandbags to prevent rotation.

Medial distraction

Place adhesive tape or a tie around the distal radius/ulna proximal to the carpus (without obscuring any of the carpal bones). Secure the tape medially (a sandbag may be useful). Place a second piece of tape around the foot and distract the distal limb laterally and secure it in the same way. Collimate to include the distal third of the radius/ulna and the foot.

Lateral distraction

Repeat as for the medial distraction view but reverse the tapes.

Comments

These stressed views are used when collateral joint instability is suspected. They can also be used to highlight suspected carpal fractures but care must be taken not to cause additional fracture displacement. It is important to include the foot as this will help to visualize the degree of laxity in the joint. Markers should be used at the level of each tape to identify the direction of forces used to stress the joint.

Carpus (2)

Views

- Mediolateral extended view
- Mediolateral flexed view

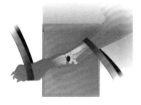
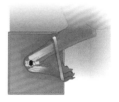

Beam centring

Centre at the level of the antebrachiocarpal joint.

Positioning and collimation

Place the patient in lateral recumbency with the limb under investigation adjacent to the cassette. The other limb should be secured caudally using a tie. Using adhesive tapes or ties proximal and distal to the carpal joint, the carpus should be secured in maximum extension for the extended view, and in maximum flexion for the flexed view. Collimate to include the distal third of the radius/ulna and the foot.

Comments

Including the foot helps to visualize the degree of laxity in the joint.

Tarsus (1)

View

- Plantarodorsal laterally and medially stressed views

Beam centring

Centre in the midline at the level of the tibiotarsal joint. ➠

Positioning and collimation

Place the patient in sternal recumbency with the head supported on a foam pad. Place padding under the hindlimb not under investigation. This helps to rotate the pelvis so that the limb of interest can be fully extended caudally. Apply adhesive tapes or ties proximal and distal to the tarsal joint, distracting the proximal limb medially and the distal limb laterally. Collimate to include the distal third of the tibia and the foot. Reverse the tapes to distract the joint medially.

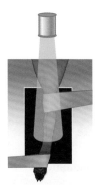

Comments

Markers should be used at the level of each tape to identify the direction of forces used to stress the joint.

Tarsus (2)

Views

- Mediolateral extended view

- Mediolateral flexed view

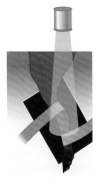

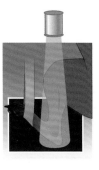

Beam centring

Centre at the level of the tibiotarsal joint.

Positioning and collimation

Place the patient in lateral recumbency with the limb under investigation adjacent to the cassette. The other limb should be secured out of the way using a tie. Apply adhesive tape or a tie proximal and distal to the tarsal joint and secure the joint in maximum extension or in maximum flexion as required. Collimate to include the distal third of the tibia and the foot.

Comments

Including the foot helps to visualize the degree of laxity in the joint.

Shoulder

View

- Cranioproximal–craniodistal oblique (CrPr–CrDiO) flexed skyline view

Beam centring

Centre over the bicipital groove between the greater and lesser tuberosities of the humerus.

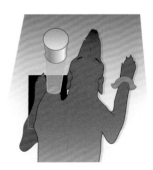

Positioning and collimation

Place the patient in sternal recumbency, with the head supported on a foam pad and rotated away from the shoulder to be radiographed. The sternum should also be rotated slightly away from the shoulder. Pads placed under the opposite forelimb may help with positioning. The limb under investigation needs to be fully flexed and the ⟶

carpus brought caudally so that it is under the shoulder, with the foot placed slightly medially. The elbow needs to be held close to the body, which will help to keep the humerus straight. The cassette needs to be positioned into the crease of the elbow, held in position between the humerus and radius. Collimate to include the area of interest.

Comments

This view is useful in the investigation of mineralized opacities seen on a mediolateral view, and helps to determine whether such opacities lie within the bicipital groove. It is also useful for showing any new bone formation within the groove.

NOTES

Recumbent patient care[16]

Parameter	Potential problems	Possible nursing interventions
Eating	Inability to eat May require a 'special' diet Inappropriate weight gain/loss	Provide palatable food Supportive feeding Provide a food appropriate for any underlying medical conditions Monitor weight regularly (daily)
Drinking	Inability to drink or inadequate water intake	Monitor water intake Assess hydration i.v. fluids as necessary
Urinating	May urinate in bedding Urine scalding and decubital ulcers	Monitor urination Take dogs outside frequently Provide appropriate bedding, including incontinence pads Urinary catheterization as necessary Monitor for urine scalding and decubital ulcers
Defecating	Defecating in bedding Constipation Diarrhoea Urine scalding and decubital ulcers	Monitor defecation carefully Take dogs outside frequently Provide appropriate bedding, including incontinence pads Provide treatments as necessary, including enemas and laxatives Keep clean Monitor carefully for urine scalding and decubital ulcers
Breathing	Underlying breathing problems Hypostatic pneumonia	Treat any existing problems Prevent and monitor for hypostatic congestion/pneumonia

Parameter	Potential problems	Possible nursing interventions
Maintaining body temperature	May be hyperthermic, normothermic or hypothermic	Monitor temperature and provide appropriate nursing care, including heat provision as required
Grooming	Coat may become soiled Urine scalding and decubital ulcers	Groom frequently Keep clean Monitor for urine scalding and decubital ulcers
Mobilizing	Unlikely to mobilize normally Prone to secondary problems (urine scalding, decubital ulcers, hypostatic pneumonia)	Turn patients at least every 4h Provide good bedding Provide appropriate physiotherapy
Sleeping/ resting	May be unsettled and have disturbed sleep May sleep during the day and have disturbed nights Nursing interventions may disturb sleep	Provide stimulation and a regular routine Provide nursing care in a way that minimizes disturbance of sleep
Expressing normal behaviour	Can become very bored	Provide encouragement and TLC Take outside if possible

NOTES

Resting energy requirement (RER) calculation[16]

The following equation can be used to calculate the RER for cats or dogs:

RER (kcal/day) = 70 x bodyweight (kg)$^{0.75}$

Alternatively, for animals weighing between 2 and 30 kg, the following linear formula gives a good approximation of energy needs:

RER (kcal/day) = 30 x bodyweight (kg) + 70

Note: To convert kcal to kilojoules (kJ) multiply by 4.185

Robert Jones bandage *see* **Bandaging**

NOTES

NOTES

Scrubbing[16]

Surgical scrub solutions

Agent	Properties
Povidone–iodine	• Iodine combined with a detergent • Broad-spectrum antimicrobial activity (bactericidal, viricidal and fungicidal) • May cause severe skin reactions and irritation in some individuals • Efficacy impaired by organic matter
Chlorhexidine	• Effective against many bacteria (including *Escherichia coli* and *Pseudomonas* spp.) • Viricidal, fungicidal and sporicidal properties • Effective level of activity in presence of organic material • Longer residual activity than povidone–iodine • Relatively low toxicity to tissue
Triclosan	• Newer agent, claimed to be antibacterial against both Gram-positive and Gram-negative bacteria

Skin preparation technique

1. Put on surgical gloves to prevent contamination of the patient's skin from the hands. It is not necessary for the gloves to be sterile during the initial preparation, although good hand hygiene should be adopted (**see Hand hygiene**).
2. Using lint-free swabs and a dilute surgical scrub solution (chlorhexidine gluconate diluted 50:50 in water), clean the site. Lint-free swabs should always be used, never cotton wool. A reasonable amount of friction is required. The site should be cleaned from the expected line of surgical incision out to the edge of the clipped area; once the edges of the clipped area are reached, without the surrounding fur being included, the swab should be discarded and a new one used.
3. Continue this procedure until the area is clean, i.e. there is no discoloration or dirt visible on a white swab.

⟶

4. Avoid over-wetting the patient. For limb surgery that does not involve the foot, it should be wrapped in a non-sterile cohesive bandage to allow for draping once transferred into the operating theatre. Care should be taken to avoid soaking the coat, as this will increase the risk of 'strike-through' from the drapes, and may make the patient hypothermic, especially in the case of small pets.

5. Cover the area with a clean sheet (kennel liners work well). Move the patient into the theatre and position for surgery. For limb surgery, a limb tie or tape is applied over the bandaged foot and attached to a transfusion stand. This allows preparation around all sides of the limb as the limb is suspended.

6. If the surgical site was contaminated in the transition to the theatre, clean the skin again in the manner previously described.

7. The final stage of preparation involves the wearing of sterile gloves and the application of an antiseptic skin solution. There are commercially available applicators containing chlorhexidine and isopropyl alcohol at the correct ratio. The manufacturers' guidelines state that these products are applied to the skin in a back and forth method. Products that are sprayed over the surgical site and allowed to dry on to the skin (e.g. chlorhexidine isopropyl), do not provide any mechanical element of cleaning.

Scrub routine

1. Remove watch and jewellery.
2. Adjust the water supply (which should be elbow- or foot-operated) to a suitable temperature and flow.
3. Wash the hands thoroughly using an antimicrobial soap, adopting a good hand washing technique (**see Hand hygiene**). At this stage, clean the nails using a nail pick.
4. Once the hands have been washed, wash the arms up to the elbows. Always keep the hands higher than

the elbows so that water drains down towards the unscrubbed upper arms. The purpose of this stage of the procedure is to remove organic matter and grease from the skin.

5. Rinse the hands and then the lower arms, allowing water to wash away the soap from the hands towards the elbows.

6. Using a surgical scrub solution begin the surgical scrub. Use only sufficient water to produce a lather, as bactericidal properties of the scrub solution are dependent on contact time with the skin. Excessive amounts of water will rinse away the scrub solution before it has achieved its aim.

7. Lather the surgical scrub solution over the arms before scrubbing the hands. Take a sterile scrubbing brush and systematically scrub the hands. Scrub the palms of the hand, wrist and four surfaces of each finger and thumb (back, front and both sides) and the nails. Either rinse the brush and use it on the other hand or discard it and take a second brush. It is not recommended that the backs of the hands and arms are scrubbed as this may lead to excoriation, which predisposes to infection.

8. When both hands have been scrubbed for the correct contact time, drop the brush into the sink. Begin to rinse the hands and arms as before, ensuring that the hands are constantly kept above the elbows to allow the water to drain away from the hands and off the elbows.

9. The final stage is to wash the hands and wrists in surgical scrub solution. This time the scrubbing process is not extended to the elbow, so there is no danger that a previously unscrubbed area is touched.

10. Rinse the hands and arms as before.

11. Take a sterile hand towel, holding it at arm's length. Use a different quarter to dry each hand and each arm. Then discard the hand towel. ▪▪▪➡

Once the scrubbing up routine has started, the hands must not touch the taps, sink or scrub dispenser. If these are inadvertently touched, the process must start again at Step 3.

Scrub routine for alcohol hand solution

1. Wash hands with a pH neutral detergent to remove gross contamination. Dry thoroughly with paper towels (non-sterile).
2. Apply the alcohol-based solution to the hands and arms, up to the elbow. Use enough for good coverage of the whole area.
3. For the first 30 seconds, the alcohol solution is applied up to the elbows; it is important that the areas remain wet with solution. For the second 30 seconds application is only up to the wrists, and for the final 30 seconds the solution is only rubbed into the hands. Care needs to be taken to include the nail beds.
4. Rub the solution into the hands until they are dry. Do not remove any of the solution with a towel or place a gown whilst the hands are still damp.

This method is not a substitute for good hand hygiene, and some basic rules must be followed in order for it to work correctly. Gross contamination must be removed from the hands prior to scrubbing, preferably with a pH neutral soap. Many people find the health of the skin of their hands improves when using this method.

Skin sampling *see* Hair and skin sampling procedures

Sterilization – packing instruments [13, 16]

- **Linen drapes**
  - **Advantages:** Readily available; conforming; can be used to pack difficult items.
  - **Disadvantages:** Porous; liable to wear; time spent laundering and folding.
  - **Type of sterilization method:** Autoclave with drying cycle or ethylene oxide if not too tightly packed.
- **Paper drapes**
  - **Advantages:** Water-resistant so useful as outer layer to package surgical kits.
  - **Disadvantages:** Non-conforming; can be torn easily.
  - **Type of sterilization method:** Autoclave with drying cycle or ethylene oxide.
- **Self-seal sterilization bags**
  - **Advantages:** Easy to pack; clear front so able to see contents.
  - **Disadvantages:** Heavier or sharp instruments may puncture bag (to prevent punctures double packing may be necessary, which increases cost).
  - **Type of sterilization method:** Autoclave or ethylene oxide.
- **Nylon films**
  - **Advantages:** Cheap; long-lasting; readily available.
  - **Disadvantages:** Punctures easily – punctures not easily seen so may be missed.
  - **Type of sterilization method:** Autoclave.
- **Metal tins**
  - **Advantages:** Easy to pack; very long-lasting after initial expense; cannot be punctured by sharp or heavy instruments.
  - **Disadvantages:** Expensive to buy; bulky to store; need a large autoclave with a drying cycle.
  - **Type of sterilization method:** Autoclave or hot-air oven.

⠀⟿

- **Special polythene bags supplied by manufacturers of ethylene oxide**
  - **Advantages:** Easy to use, strong bags.
  - **Disadvantages:** Must use specific polythene bags with correct equipment; can overpack so gas cannot circulate.
  - **Type of sterilization method:** Ethylene oxide.
- **Cardboard cartons**
  - **Advantages:** Sturdy and not easily punctured by sharp objects; regular shape makes them neat to store.
  - **Disadvantages:** Expensive to buy; can be bulky to store.
  - **Type of sterilization method:** Autoclave with drying cycle.

See also **Folding gowns and drapes**

NOTES

Sterilization indicators [13, 16]

Method	Comments	Use with
Chemical indicator strips	Show a colour change when exposed to the correct conditions. Should be placed in centre of pack before sterilization	
	• Chemical indicator strips: paper strips that change colour when exposed to correct conditions of temperature, pressure and time; also available for ethylene oxide	Autoclave, ethylene oxide
	• Browne's tube: small glass tube filled with orange liquid that changes to green when correct temperature is reached and maintained for correct length of time. Available for different temperatures	Autoclave, hot-air oven
Indicator tape	Often used as method of securing other packing materials. Tape only indicates exposure, not that correct time or pressure has been achieved; therefore cannot be considered as reliable method for checking sterilization	
	• Bowie Dick tape: beige with series of lines on it that change to black after exposure to temperature of 121°C	Autoclave
	• Ethylene oxide tape: green with series of lines that change to red after exposure to ethylene oxide gas	Ethylene oxide
Spore strips	Paper strips that contain a controlled-count spore population. After sterilization, strips are cultured for 72 hours to see if all spores destroyed. Main disadvantage is delay in obtaining results	Autoclave, hot-air oven, ethylene oxide

NOTES

Surgical checklist[16]

The surgical safety checklist has been incorporated in many veterinary operating theatres. Guidelines from the World Health Organization (WHO) provide examples and can be used to create a checklist relevant to the practice (www.who.int/patientsafety/safesurgery/checklist/en/). The checklists are split into preoperative and postoperative sections and are used to introduce the team, record items opened on to the instrument trolley, record any anticipated critical events and discuss any concerns relating to the patient.

The preoperative checklist is read out and completed by the circulating nurse, after draping but prior to the first incision. It is important that all members of the team stop completely for this brief period of time for full concentration. Any anticipated critical events can be discussed and a plan made for what to do in these situations.

See also **Anaesthetic checklists**

NOTES

Before anaesthesia

(at least nurse)

Confirm:

☐ Patient identity
☐ Procedure
☐ Consent form signed

Check:

☐ Medications given
☐ Anaesthetic machine
☐ Ancillary surgical equipment
☐ Instruments sterilized

Date:

Signed:

Before surgical incision

(all theatre staff)

☐ **Team have introduced themselves**

Confirm:

☐ Patient identity
☐ Procedure
☐ Suitability of clip
☐ Bladder empty (abdominal operations)
☐ Specific preoperative preparations
☐ Antibiosis if required
☐ Other perioperative medication

Anticipated critical steps

Surgeon:

☐ What are the critical steps?
☐ Anticipated time to completion

Anaesthetist/nurse:

☐ Anaesthetic-specific concerns

Nurse/surgical assistant:

☐ Sterility of instruments
☐ Any equipment concerns
☐ Essential radiographs displayed

Before leaving theatre

(at least surgeon and nurse)

Nurse verbally confirms:

☐ Swab count
☐ Sharps accounted for
☐ Specimen labelling *(read aloud)*

☐ Any equipment issues to be addressed

What are the key concerns for recovery and postoperative management?

Specific medication and care

Notes: *(turn over if needed)*

Veterinary surgery safety checklist, modified form the World Health Organization (WHO) surgical safety checklist. (© Romain Pizzi, Zoological Medicine Ltd)

Sutures[12, 13, 16]

Absorbable suture materials

Suture material	Trade name	Mono/multi-filament	Synthetic/natural	Coated	
Polyglactin 910	Vicryl (Ethicon) Polysorb (USSC)	Multi (braided)	Synthetic	Yes (calcium stearate)	
Polydioxanone	PDS II (Ethicon)	Mono	Synthetic	No	
Polyglycolic acid	Dexon (USSC)	Multi	Synthetic	Can be coated with polymers	
Poliglecaprone 25	Monocryl (Ethicon) Caprosyn (USSC)	Mono	Synthetic	No	

NOTES

Duration of strength	Absorption	Comments/uses
Retains 50% of tensile strength at 14 days, 20% at 21 days	Absorption 60–90 days by hydrolysis	Dyed or undyed Low tissue reactivity Uses: subcutis, muscle, eyes, hollow viscera
Retains 70% tensile strength at 14 days, 14% at 56 days	Only minimal absorption by 90 days, absorbed by 180 days Absorbed by hydrolysis	Good for infected sites as monofilament Very strong but springy Minimal tissue reaction Uses: subcutis, muscle, sometimes eyes
Retains 20% at 14 days	Complete absorption by 100–120 days Absorbed by hydrolysis	Similar to polyglactin but has considerable tissue drag Uses: as for polyglactin
Retains approximately 60% at 7 days, 30% at 14 days Wound support maintained for 20 days	Complete absorption between 90 and 120 days Absorbed by hydrolysis	Less springy than other monofilament absorbables with minimal tissue reaction and drag Available dyed or undyed

NOTES

Non-absorbable suture materials

Suture material	Trade name	Mono- or multi-filament	Synthetic/ natural	Coated	
Polyamide (nylon)	Ethilon (Ethicon), Monosof (USSC)	Mono	Synthetic	No	
Polybutester	Novafil (Davis & Geck)	Mono	Synthetic	No	
Polypropylene	Prolene (Ethicon), Surgipro (USSC)	Mono	Synthetic	No	
Braided silk	Mersilk (Ethicon)	Multi	Natural	Wax coat	
Braided polyamide	Supramid or Nurolon (Ethicon)	Multi	Synthetic	Encased in outer sheath	
Surgical stainless steel wire		Available as either mono or multi	Synthetic	No	

NOTES

Knot security	Duration	Comments
Fair	Permanent	Causes minimal tissue reaction and has little tissue drag
Fair	Permanent	Very similar to Ethilon, with similar properties
Fair, can produce bulky knots that untie easily	Permanent	Very inert, produces only minimal tissue reaction Very strong but also very springy Little tissue drag
Excellent	Eventually may fragment and break down	Natural material with good handling properties but high tissue reactivity and should not be used in infected sites
Good	Outer sheath can be broken	Better handling characteristics than monofilament polyamide Can be used in the skin but should not be used as buried suture
Excellent but knots may be difficult to tie	Permanent	Not commonly used now but can be useful in bone or tendon Difficult to handle, may break

NOTES

Suture patterns

Continuous

Simple continuous (SC)

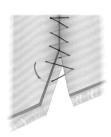

- Description: Running stitch.
- Particular features: Rapidly placed; prone to patient interference if used in skin; theoretically insecure.
- Typical application: Fascia, including midline; muscle; viscera.

Intradermal/subcuticular

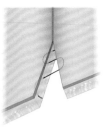

- Description: Buried continuous stitch to close skin.
- Particular features: Slower than other skin patterns; resists tension; avoids patient interference; does not require removal.
- Typical application: Skin; presence of tension; sites prone to interference (e.g. castration).

Interrupted

Simple interrupted appositional (SIA)

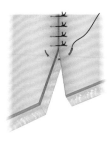

- Description: Individual stitches placed as simple loops across wound.
- Particular features: The standard pattern; produces good apposition.
- Typical application: Skin closure; midline closure; viscera closure.

Horizontal mattress

- Description: Placed as loops with a bite on each side of wound parallel to wound edge.
- Particular features: Produces some eversion; resists effects of tension more than SIA.
- Typical application: Skin, especially in presence of tension.

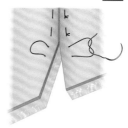

Cruciate mattress

- Description: Similar to horizontal mattress but strands cross over wound.
- Particular features: Less eversion than above; resists effects of tension more than SIA; faster than above.
- Typical application: Skin, especially in presence of tension.

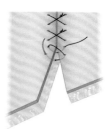

Vertical mattress

- Description: Placed as loops with a bite on each side of wound perpendicular to wound edge.
- Particular features: Produces some eversion; resists effects of tension more than SIA; interferes with blood supply less than horizontal mattress.
- Typical application: Skin, especially in presence of tension; most commonly used interspersed with SIA to resist effects of tension.

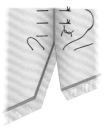

NOTES

Temperature conversion[16]

Temperature conversion

To convert Celsius to Fahrenheit – multiply by 9, divide by 5 and add 32. For example 38.5°C = 101.3°F:

- 38.5°C x 9 = 346.5
- $\dfrac{346.5}{5}$ = 69.3
- 69.3 + 32 = 101.3°F

To convert Fahrenheit to Celsius – subtract 32, multiply by 5 and divide by 9. For example 102.5°F = 39.2°C:

- 102.5°F – 32 = 70.5
- 70.5 x 5 = 352.5
- $\dfrac{352.5}{9}$ = 39.2°C

NOTES

Theatre – maintenance of asepsis[16]

- Correct theatre attire should be worn at all times.
- There should be the minimum number of people required present within the operating theatre; movement should be kept to a minimum and all doors closed.
- There should be a new set of sterile instruments for each operation, even when dealing with a contaminated site. More than one set may be required to prevent tumour seeding or contamination.
- There should be a plan to perform 'clean' operations first in the day, and to carry out contaminated surgery last.
- Wherever possible there should be separate rooms for 'dirty' and 'clean' procedures.
- An efficient sterilization programme should be adopted.
- The theatre should be maintained at an ambient temperature (18–21°C) and the ventilation must be good (a minimum of 20 air changes per hour). Hot, humid conditions encourage the growth of pathogens, in particular *Pseudomonas* spp.
- Patients should be clipped and have an initial skin preparation performed before they are taken to theatre.
- The surgical team must ensure that they do not touch any non-sterile surfaces during surgery. Any break in asepsis must be reported and rectified.
- No contaminated instruments or equipment should be returned to the sterile trolley.
- Good hand hygiene is required before touching a patient, before a clean or aseptic procedure, after touching a patient, after handling bodily fluids and after touching a patient's surroundings.
- Sterile gloves should be worn for all aseptic procedures.
- A record of all surgical procedures should be kept, so that if any sepsis problems arise the cause can be detected.

- A strict cleaning protocol must be maintained.
- Dedicated equipment should be available for surgical procedures, which is appropriately maintained and sterilized.

***See also* Cleaning the operating theatre**

NOTES

Total solids — using a refractometer[16]

Measuring total solids using a refractometer

1. Prepare and measure PCV on a microhaematocrit tube (**see Packed cell volume — how to perform a PCV**).
2. Ensure that the refractometer is calibrated (see Step 6, below).
3. Carefully break the capillary tube near the bottom of the plasma fraction. This will give two fragments, one containing the plasma and the other the packed cells.

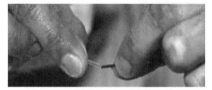

4. Discard the packed cells fragment into a sharps bin.
5. Dab the unbroken end of the fragment containing the plasma on to the refractometer surface. Be careful not to cut yourself on the sharp edges of the glass.

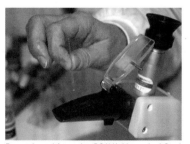

Reproduced from the *BSAVA Manual of Canine and Feline Clinical Pathology, 3rd edn*

6. Read the appropriate scale on the refractometer to determine the plasma protein; this is usually the left hand scale and may be labelled 'Serum P'.

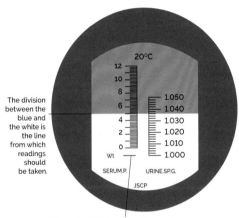

The division between the blue and the white is the line from which readings should be taken.

When only distilled water is placed on to the reading plate, the line should appear at this point if properly calibrated.

7. The measurement will be g/100 ml so needs to be multiplied by 10 to give g/litre (e.g. 50 g/litre above).
8. Dispose of the remaining glass into a sharps bin.

NOTES

Urinalysis[13]

Summary of tests

VISUAL INSPECTION

Assess colour and turbidity (cloudiness)

SPECIFIC GRAVITY (SG)

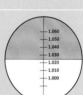

1. To calibrate refractometer, place distilled water beneath plastic cover of refractometer.
2. Adjust until SG = 1.000 and then dry refractometer.
3. Place urine under plastic cover of refractometer.
4. Read SG (the point where red area turns to white; in the example (right) the SG is 1.024).
5. Rinse and dry refractometer.

Note: Dipstick assessment of SG is inaccurate

DIPSTICK ANALYSIS (pH, glucose, ketones, protein, bilirubin)

1. Invert urine sample to ensure thorough mixing.
2. Cover all squares on dipstick with urine and note time.
3. Read dipstick results at times indicated on barrel.

Note: Dipstick SG is inaccurate and dipsticks will not detect all types of ketones

MICROSCOPIC EXAMINATION OF SEDIMENT

Examine as soon as possible after collection

1. Centrifuge 10 ml at 2000 rpm for 5 minutes.
2. Remove supernatant and resuspend sediment by tapping tube.

Wet preparation:

- Place a drop of suspension on a slide and stain with new methylene blue if necessary
- Place a coverslip over the urine

Dry preparation:

- Make a smear using a drop of resuspended sediment
- Rapidly air-dry and stain with Leishman's stain

Microscopic appearance of common urinary crystals

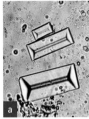
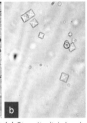
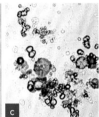

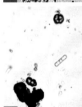

(a) Struvite (triple phosphate) crystals.
(b) Calcium oxalate crystals. (c) Calcium carbonate crystals. (d) Ammonium nitrate crystals.

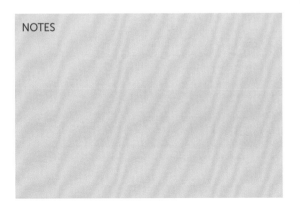

NOTES

U

Urinary catheters – cats [13, 16]

Type	Photograph	Sex	Material	Indwelling	Sizes (FG)	Length (cm)	Luer fitting
Plastic cat catheter		Male and female	Flexible grade of nylon	No	3 and 4	30.5	Yes
Jackson cat catheter		Male and female	Flexible grade of nylon	Yes	3 and 4	11	Yes
Silicone cat catheter		Male	Medical grade silicone	Yes	3.5	12	Yes
Slippery Sam™ catheter		Male	PTFE (Teflon™)	Yes	3–3.5	14 and 11	Yes

Types of urinary catheter suitable for cats. FG = French gauge

Catheterizing a tomcat

Equipment
As for dog catheterization (see page 241).

Restraint
The cat should usually be sedated and positioned in lateral recumbency with the hindlimbs pulled slightly cranially. The tail should be held away from the perineal area.

Procedure
1. Wash your hands and put on gloves.
2. Prepare the feeding sleeve as for the dog catheter and lubricate the tip (see page 241).
3. With one hand, extrude the penis by applying gentle pressure each side of the prepuce with two fingers.
4. Introduce the catheter into the urethra gently.
5. Collect the sample or drain the bladder.
6. If a Jackson catheter is being placed for continuous drainage, stitch the flange to the prepuce.

Catheterizing a queen

Equipment
As for dog catheterization (see page 243).

Restraint
The cat should usually be sedated and positioned in lateral recumbency with the hindlimbs pulled slightly cranially. The tail should be held away from the perineal area.

Procedure
1. Wash your hands and put on gloves.
2. Remove the outer wrapping and cut a feeding sleeve.
3. Lubricate the tip of the catheter.
4. Place the catheter between the vulval lips and 'blindly' introduce it into the urethra. Angle the catheter ventrally, placing gentle pressure until the catheter slips into the urethra.
5. The catheter is not designed to be indwelling.

Urinary catheters — dogs[13, 16]

Type	Photograph	Sex	Material	Indwelling	Sizes (FG)	Length (cm)	Luer fitting
Plastic dog catheter		Male and female	Flexible grade of nylon (polyamide)	No but can be adapted to be indwelling	6–10	50–60	Yes
Foley		Female	Teflon-coated latex	Yes	8–16	30–40	No
Silicone Foley		Male and female	Flexible medical grade silicone	Yes	5–10	30 and 55	No
Tieman's		Female	PVC (polyvinyl chloride)	No	8–12	43	Yes

Types of urinary catheter suitable for dogs. FG = French gauge

Catheterizing a male dog

Equipment

- Catheter
- Swabs for cleaning
- Sterile water-based lubricant (or silicone spray)
- Syringe to assist urine drainage
- Three-way tap (if required)
- Sample pot
- Gloves
- Urine bag or a bung
- Kidney dish

If the catheter is to be made indwelling, the following equipment is also required:

- Suture material
- Zinc oxide tape
- For silicone male Foley catheters, water sufficient to fill balloon
- Guide wire
- Syringe.

Restraint

Dogs may be restrained in a standing position or in lateral recumbency.

Procedure

1. Wash your hands and put on gloves.
2. Clean the prepuce.
3. Extrude the penis; if not experienced, ask an assistant to do this.
4. Clean the prepuce again.
5. Remove the catheter 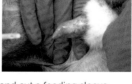 from the outer wrapping and cut a feeding sleeve from the inner sterile packaging. This allows easy feeding of the catheter from the packaging into the urethra using a 'no touch' technique.

▰▰▰➡

For silicone male Foley catheter placement, feed the guide wire up the centre of the catheter.

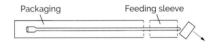

6. Lubricate the catheter and insert the tip into the urethra.
7. Advance the catheter up the urethra. Resistance may be met at the os penis, where there is a slight narrowing of the urethra, at the ischial arch and at the area of the prostate gland if enlarged. Steady but gentle pressure should overcome this resistance. If the catheter cannot be passed, re-evaluate catheter size.
8. Inflate the balloon once the tip of the catheter is in the bladder if using a silicone male Foley.
9. Proceed according to the reason for catheterization (e.g. drain bladder, collect sample, hydropropulsion).

To make an indwelling dog catheter from a polyamide catheter, either:

■ Place zinc tape around the catheter near to the prepuce

OR

■ Stitch or stick the catheter to the prepuce.

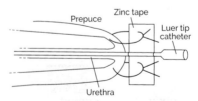

Neither of these options is ideal because dog catheters are not designed to be indwelling. It is best to use a silicone indwelling male Foley.

Catheterizing a bitch

Method 1: Urethra viewed in dorsal recumbency

Equipment
- Speculum (with or without light source)
- Alternative light source if required
- Catheter
- Sterile water-based lubricant (or silicone spray)
- Swabs for cleaning
- Gloves

If a Foley catheter is being placed, the following equipment is also needed:

- Stylet
- Sterile water/saline to inflate cuff
- Urine bag
- Syringe.

Restraint
Bitches should usually be sedated for this procedure. The bitch should be positioned in a straight dorsal recumbent position with the hindlimbs flexed and drawn forward. The tail must also be under control.

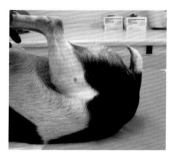

⸫⟶

Procedure

1. Wash your hands and put on gloves.
2. Clean the vulva.
3. Remove the catheter from its outer wrapping and expose the tip only from the inner sleeve.
4. If a Foley catheter is being used, insert the stylet.
5. Place the lubricated speculum blades between the vulval lips as caudally as possible to avoid the clitoral fossa.

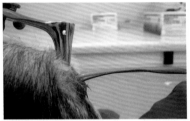

6. Insert vertically into the vestibule and turn the handles cranially.
7. Open the blades of the speculum. The urethral opening will be visible on the cranial side of the vertically oriented vestibule, approximately half way between the vulva and cervix.

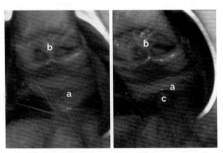

a = the urethral orifice; **b** = clitoral fossa; **c** = catheter in position.

8. Insert the tip of the catheter into the urethral orifice. Draw the hindlimbs caudally. This straightens the urethra, making it easier to push the catheter into the bladder.

9. Proceed depending on the reason for catheterization. If a Foley catheter is being used, inflate the balloon, withdraw the stylet, attach the urine collecting bag and place an Elizabethan collar.

Method 2: Urethra viewed standing

Equipment

The equipment required is as for Method 1. Generally only one assistant is required.

Restraint

The bitch should generally be standing for this procedure, although positioned in a straight ventral recumbency with the hindlimbs forwards is also possible. Ensure the tail is well restrained.

Procedure

1. Wash your hands and put on gloves.
2. Clean the vulva.
3. Place the speculum between the vulval lips and advance at a slight angle towards the spine, then horizontally.
4. Open the blades and identify the urethral orifice. This will be on the ventral floor of the vestibule.
5. Insert the catheter at a slightly ventral angle so as to follow the direction of the urethra into the bladder.
6. Proceed as for Method 1.

Method 3: Digital

Equipment

- Sterile gloves
- Catheter
- Sterile water-based lubricant (or silicone spray)
- Swabs for cleaning
- Collection pots

If a Foley catheter is being placed, the additional equipment required is as for Method 1.

Restraint

The bitch should generally be standing for this procedure, although lateral recumbency is also possible.

Procedure

1. Scrub your hands and put on sterile gloves in an aseptic manner.
2. Ask an assistant to clean the vulva.
3. The assistant removes the outer wrapping from the catheter and you (the scrubbed person) remove the inner package.
4. Holding the sterile part of the packaging, place the stylet if necessary.
5. Lubricate the first finger of your non-writing hand.
6. Place your finger into the vestibule and feel along the ventral surface for a raised pimple.
7. Place your finger just cranial to this raised area, which is the urethral orifice.

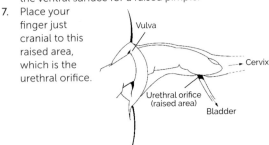

8. Raising your hand and finger dorsally, digitally guide the catheter, tipped slightly ventrally (as for Method 2) into the urethral orifice. The catheter will run past the fingertip if the orifice is missed.

9. Proceed as for Method 1.

The digital method may be difficult or even impossible in smaller breeds.

NOTES

Urine specific gravity (USG) normal values[13]

- Dog 1.015–1.040
- Cat 1.015–1.050
- Rabbit 1.003–1.036

There can be variation from these ranges, depending on the age, breed, sex and hydration status of the animal.

NOTES

Velpeau sling *see* **Bandaging**

Vernier scale[13]

Each scale on a microscope consists of a main scale divided into millimetres and a Vernier plate with 10 divisions. Vernier scales can be used to record the location of a particular part of an image or specimen, so that it can be relocated easily on subsequent viewing. There are two scales: the horizontal Vernier scale (X axis running from left to right) and the vertical Vernier scale (Y axis running from top to bottom). Both must be read and recorded, stating horizontal and vertical values (X, Y).

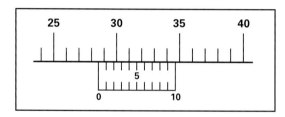

1. Observe where the division labelled 'zero' on the plate meets the main scale. If it falls between two divisions, record the lower number (28).
2. Note which of the plate divisions is aligned with a mark on the main scale (4).
3. The reading is recorded as the first number with the second number after the point (28.4).
4. Repeat the reading for the scale at right angles.
5. The readings are reported in same way as grid references on a map.

Always place the slide with the label to the right so that points can be relocated.

Vital signs — normal ranges in common species

Species	Body temperature (°C)	Heart rate (beats/min)	Respiratory rate (breaths/min)
Dog	38.3–39.2	70–140	10–30
Cat	38.2–38.6	100–200	20–30
Ferret	37.8–40	200–250	33–36
Domestic rabbit	38.5–40	130–325	30–60
Chinchilla	37–38	200–350	40–80
Guinea pig	37.2–39.5	230–380	90–150
Chipmunk	38 (during torpor, a few degrees above ambient)	264–296 (during torpor, may drop to 3–6)	75 (during torpor, may drop to <1 and is barely detectable)
Gerbil	37.4–39	260–600	85–160
Hamster (Russian)	36–38	300–460	60–80
Hamster (Syrian)	36.2–37.5	300–470	40–110
Rat	38	310–500	70–150
Mouse	37.5	420–700	100–250

NOTES

Wound drain management[13]

- Use aseptic techniques for all postoperative drain care.
- Clip a large area of hair around the wound, especially the area dependent to the wound.
- Use petroleum jelly or barrier spray to protect the skin dependent to the drain exit hole from maceration.
- Clean the exposed drain and skin exit holes twice daily with an antiseptic solution, such as povidone–iodine.
- Empty and change active suction devices as often as required to maintain function.
- Cover with a sterile dressing and light bandage. Change as often as necessary to prevent wound fluid penetrating to the outer dressing layer (strikethrough) and to maintain asepsis.
- Prevent patient interference with the drain.
- Drains are kept in place no longer than necessary, typically 2–5 days, until drainage has almost ceased. Some fluid will always be produced by a wound with a drain due to tissue reaction to the drain itself. The risks of complications increase with the time for which the drain is in place.

Complications of using drains include:

- Wound infection
- Wound dehiscence
- Early loss or removal from wound
- Failure of drainage
- Irritation and pain
- Drain tract cellulitis.

NOTES

Wound dressings[13, 16]

Dry

Dry-to-dry

- **Description:** Sterile gauze swabs.
- **Characteristics:** Dry swabs placed on wound to absorb exudates. Adheres to necrotic tissue.
- **Indications:**
  - Exuding wounds
  - Necrotic wounds
  - Not recommended on granulating wounds.

Wet-to-dry

- **Description:** Sterile gauze swabs soaked in sterile saline.
- **Characteristics:** Dry swabs soaked in sterile saline applied on wound. Adheres to necrotic tissue.
- **Indications:**
  - Exuding wounds
  - Necrotic wounds
  - Not recommended on granulating wounds.

Non-adherent – 1

- **Description:** Perforated polyester film, absorbent 80% cotton 20% viscose pad, non-woven backing material.
- **Characteristics:** Shiny side down on wound. Does not absorb exudates and can adhere to exuding wounds. Needs secondary dressings.
- **Examples:** Melolin (Smith & Nephew), Primapore (Smith & Nephew).
- **Indications:**
  - Dry wounds
  - Postoperative wounds
  - Sutures.

Non-adherent – 2

- **Description:** Bleached cotton/rayon cloth impregnated with white or yellow soft paraffin.

- **Characteristics:** Paraffin reduces adherence to wound but can dry out if not changed regularly. Needs secondary dressing.
- **Examples:** Jelonet (Smith & Nephew), Grassolind (Millpledge).
- Indications:
  - Clean superficial wounds
  - Abrasions
  - Cuts.

Interactive
Hydrogels

- **Description:** 2.3% modified sodium carboxymethylcellulose polymer, 77.7% water, 20% propylene glycol, 3.5% starch grafted polymer aqueous base, 20% propylene glycol.
- **Characteristics:** Available as flat sheets or gels. Have high water content; can rehydrate wounds and ensure moist wound healing. Cool surface of wound. Too much can cause maceration. Can be mixed with topical medications. Need secondary dressing.
  Examples: IntraSite (Smith & Nephew), Manuka (Kruuse), Activon Tulle (Advancis).
- Indications:
  - Desloughing
  - Exuding wounds
  - Abscess cavities.

Hydrocolloids

- **Description:** Microgranular suspension of polymers – consists of a waterproof polyurethane foam bonded on a polyurethane film that acts as carrier for hydrocolloid base.
- **Characteristics:** Absorbs exudates into foam, leading to change in the dressing. Should be 2 cm or more either side of the wound edges. Does not require a secondary dressing.
- **Examples:** Granuflex (ConvaTec), Tegaderm (3M).
- **Indications:** Light to medium exuding wounds.

Foam

- **Description:** Absorbent polyurethane containing either hydrocellular or hydropolymer foam and some carbon. Comes in a variety of forms.
- **Characteristics:** Can absorb 6–10 times own weight in exudates. Conforms to cavity. White surface placed on wound. Exudate does not leak through. Works by capillary action drawing exudates from wound. Needs secondary dressings. Can be left in place for up to 7 days.
- **Examples:** Allevyn (Smith & Nephew), Tegaderm Foam Adhesive Dressing (3M).
- **Indications:**
  - Suitable for all types of wounds that have light to heavy exudates
  - Deep cavity wounds.

Alginate

- **Description:** Made from a variety of seaweeds, some contain calcium. Mixed into a non-woven dressing.
- **Characteristics:** Highly absorbent; dressings turn to gel once mixed with exudates. Some have haemostatic properties. Needs secondary dressings. Can be left in place for up to 7 days.
- **Examples:** Algisite M (Smith & Nephew), Kaltostat (ConvaTec).
- **Indications:**
  - Infected wounds
  - Exuding wounds
  - Cavities
  - Haemorrhage.

Collagen

- **Description:** Collagen matrix.
- **Characteristics:** Binds blood clotting factors XII and XIII. Causes natural wound cleansing. Attracts granulocytes and fibroblasts to the wound and forms an organized structure for basal cells of epidermis.

- **Example:** Vet BioSISt (Smiths-SurgiVet).
- **Indications:**
  - Most types of wounds
  - Not recommended for full thickness burns or necrotic wounds.

Silver-coated dressings

- **Description:** SILCRYST; nanocrystals.
- **Characteristics:** Silver ions released into wound bed have anti-inflammatory action and kill bacteria rapidly.
- **Examples:** Acticoat (Smith & Nephew).
- **Indications:** Infected wounds.

Vapour-permeable film

- **Description:** Thin conformable adhesive film.
- **Characteristics:** Provides thin vapour-permeable film, allowing vapour exchange and maintenance of moist wound environment.
- **Examples:** Opsite Flexigrid (Smith & Nephew), Tegaderm (3M).
- **Indications:**
  - Uninfected shallow wounds
  - Intact skin at risk of pressure or maceration injury.

Barrier film

- **Description:** Spray or foam containing polymer.
- **Characteristics:** Sprayed over wound; dries to leave film of polymer that is permeable to moisture vapour and air. Creates a barrier.
- **Examples:** Opsite (Smith & Nephew), Cavilon (3M).
- **Indications:**
  - Minor wounds
  - Abrasions
  - Sutures
  - Wound covering on reptiles.

Topical

Antiseptics

- **Description:** Dilute chlorhexidine 0.05%; dilute povidone–iodine 1%.
- **Characteristics:** Used for initial cleansing of wounds. These solutions can be toxic to fibroblasts and should be avoided if possible. Contaminated wounds would be better treated with debridement.
- **Examples:** Hibitane, Pevidine, antiseptic solution.
- **Indications:** Contaminated wounds.

Aloe vera

- **Description:** Gel.
- **Characteristics:** Promotes wound healing by accelerating formation of granulation tissue. Stabilizes fibroblast growth factors and activates macrophages.
- **Indications:** All wounds.

Hydrophilic cream

- **Description:** Hydrophilic cream containing silver sulfadiazine.
- **Characteristics:** Inhibits growth of bacteria and fungi *in vitro*. Studies have been carried out to show antibacterial action against meticillin-resistant *Staphylococcus aureus*, *Pseudomonas* spp. and enterococci. Cream must be placed in wound as it will macerate surrounding skin.
- **Examples:** Flamazine (Smith & Nephew).
- **Indications:** Burn wounds and wounds infected with Gram-negative bacteria.

Sugar paste and honey

- **Description:** Paste. Caster sugar and additive-free icing sugar dissolved in hydrogen peroxide and polyethylene glycol 400 has been developed for clinical use.
- **Characteristics:** Has been used in wounds for centuries. Paste has lower pH than wound and helps

to debride infected or dirty wounds. Not suitable for granulating wounds. Honey must be sterile; has a high osmotic pressure and helps to draw out exudate.
- **Indications:** Infected dirty wounds.

NOTES

Wound recognition and treatment [10]

Wound type	Description	Treatment considerations
Abrasion	Superficial wound involving destruction of varying depths of skin by friction or shearing forces. Usually bleeds minimally	When associated with a fracture, normal skin barrier is incompetent – treat fracture as grade I open
Avulsion	Characterized by tearing of tissues from attachments and creation of skin flaps. Limb avulsion injuries with extensive skin loss are called 'degloving'	Blood supply to skin may be compromised, leading to skin necrosis 2–5 days after injury. Repeat examinations and consider secondary debridement
Bite wound	A wound received from the teeth of an animal. Can cause a combination of puncture wounds, penetrating trauma, tears and crushing of tissue	Serious haemorrhage can occur if major vessels are pierced. Infection can occur from the pathogens in the biter's mouth
Burn – chemical	Direct exposure to noxious chemicals	Copious lavage to remove chemical. Ensure animal cannot lick area and ingest harmful substances
Burn – thermal	May see reddened, crusted or blackened skin. Burn injuries around the head and neck may compromise respiration	Beware of systemic complications of the burn. Attend to analgesia and cooling the area
Contusion	Blunt trauma may cause blood to pool in the subcutaneous tissue	Application of cold and analgesics. Beware of compartment syndrome
Crushing injuries	Combination of other injuries with extensive damage and contusion to the skin and deeper tissues	Assess neurological and vascular supply prior to treatment

Gunshots	These are contaminated. The heat generated in firing a bullet does not render it sterile. Open fractures may be present	Remove metal if encountered but not usually necessary to remove all fragments unless intra-articular or impinging on major structures such as nerves and arteries. Antibiosis for severe or intra-articular injuries. 'Treat the wound not the weapon'
Laceration	Created by tearing, which damages the skin and underlying tissues and may be superficial or deep and have irregular edges	Debridement and primary closure may be used if treatment is early
Penetrating foreign body	Foreign bodies such as sticks and glass can fragment, causing widespread contamination	May need extensive exploration to remove all fragments (90% of glass shards show on radiographs). Protruding foreign bodies should be left in place for transport but can be cut 2–3 cm from the body wall to minimize further internal damage by preventing the protruding shaft acting as a fulcrum
Penetrating trauma (e.g. stabbing)	Penetrating trauma is an injury that occurs when an object pierces the skin and enters a tissue of the body, creating an open wound. There may be an entry and exit hole	If abdominal or thoracic wound, check vital signs as there may be significant haemorrhage. Penetrating abdominal wounds require exploratory laparotomy
Puncture wound	A puncture wound is caused by an object piercing the skin and creating a small hole, which can be closed over and be barely visible. There is no exit wound. Damage can be superficial or deep	Infection may occur as the small puncture in the skin rapidly seals over. To treat the injury, the hole may need to be enlarged and opened, and the wound may need exploration for a foreign body such as a splinter

NOTES

NOTES

NOTES

References

1. *BSAVA Guide to Pain Management in Small Animal Practice* (2019), ed. I. Self

2. *BSAVA Guide to Procedures in Small Animal Practice, 2nd edn* (2014), ed. N. Bexfield and K. Lee

3. *BSAVA Guide to Radiographic Positioning* (2018)

4. *BSAVA Manual of Canine and Feline Advanced Veterinary Nursing, 2nd edn* (2008), ed. A. Hotston Moore and S. Rudd

5. *BSAVA Manual of Canine and Feline Anaesthesia and Analgesia, 3rd edn* (2016), ed. T. Duke-Novakovski, M. de Vries and C. Seymour

6. *BSAVA Manual of Canine and Feline Cardiorespiratory Medicine, 2nd edn* (2010), ed. V. Luis Fuentes, L.R. Johnson and S. Dennis

7. *BSAVA Manual of Canine and Feline Clinical Pathology, 3rd edn* (2016), ed. E. Villiers and J. Ristić

8. *BSAVA Manual of Canine and Feline Dentistry and Oral Surgery, 4th edn* (2018), ed. A.M. Reiter and M. Gracis

9. *BSAVA Manual of Canine and Feline Dermatology, 3rd edn* (2012), ed. H.A. Jackson and R. Marsella

10. *BSAVA Manual of Canine and Feline Emergency and Critical Care, 3rd edn* (2018), ed. L.G. King and A. Boag

11. *BSAVA Manual of Canine and Feline Radiography and Radiology* (2013), ed. A. Holloway and J.F. McConnell

12. *BSAVA Manual of Canine and Feline Surgical Principles* (2012), ed. S.J. Baines, V. Lipscomb and T. Hutchinson

13. *BSAVA Manual of Practical Veterinary Nursing* (2007), ed. E. Mullineaux and M. Jones

14. *BSAVA Manual of Small Animal Practice Management and Development* (2012), ed. C.J. Clarke and M. Chapman

15. *BSAVA Pocketbook for Vets, 2nd edn* (2019), ed. S. Middleton

16. *BSAVA Textbook of Veterinary Nursing, 6th edn* (2020), ed. B. Cooper, E. Mullineaux and L. Turner

17. *BSAVA/SAMSoc Guide to Responsible Use of Antibacterials: PROTECT ME.* Available at: www.bsavalibrary.com/protectme

18. Fletcher DJ, Boller M, Brainard BM *et al.* (2012) RECOVER evidence and knowledge gap analysis on veterinary CPR. Part 7: clinical guidelines. *Journal of Veterinary Emergency and Critical Care* **22**, S102–S131

19. Keating SCJ, Thomas AA, Flecknell PA and Leach MC (2012) Evaluation of EMLA cream for preventing pain during tattooing of rabbits: Changes in physiological, behavioural and facial expression responses. *PLOS ONE* **7**, e44437

20. Written by Emma Gerrard

21. *WSAVA (2020) Global Nutrition Guidelines.* Available at: https://wsava.org/global-guidelines/global-nutrition-guidelines

ALWAYS read the relevant monographs

Cardiac emergencies

- **Asystole or pulseless electrical activity**
  - Adrenaline: 10 µg (micrograms)/kg i.v every 3–5 minutes until return of spontaneous circulation – this is equivalent to 1 ml/10 kg using 1:10,000 concentration (100 µg/ml). Double dose if used intratracheally.
- **Hyperkalaemic myocardial toxicity**
  - Calcium: 50–150 mg/kg calcium (boro)gluconate = 0.5–1.5 ml/kg of a 10% solution i.v. over 20–30 min *or* Soluble insulin: 0.5 IU/kg i.v. followed by 2–3 g of dextrose/unit of insulin (for urinary tract obstruction but not hypoadrenocorticism). Half the dextrose should be given as a bolus and the remainder administered i.v. over 4–6h.
- **Other bradyarrhythmias**
  - Atropine: 0.01–0.03 mg/kg i.v. – this is equivalent to 0.3–1 ml/20 kg using 0.6 mg/ml solution.
- **Ventricular tachycardia**
  - Lidocaine:
  Dogs: 2–8 mg/kg i.v. in 2 mg/kg boluses, followed by a constant rate i.v. infusion of 0.025–0.1 mg/kg/min.
  Cats: 0.25–2.0 mg/kg i.v. slowly in 0.25–0.5 mg/kg boluses followed by a constant rate i.v. infusion of 0.01–0.04 mg/kg/min.

Pulmonary emergencies

- **Respiratory arrest**
  - Doxapram: 5–10 mg/kg i.v., repeat according to need; duration of effect is approximately 15–20 min. Neonates: 1–2 drops under the tongue (oral solution) or 0.1 ml i.v. into the umbilical vein; this should be used only once.